Gluten

Is it Making you Sick or Overweight?

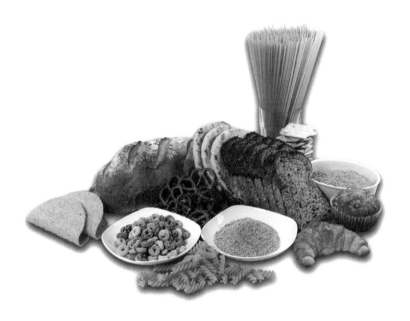

Published by
2027 W Rose Garden Lane
Phoenix, AZ 85027

Ph +1 623 334 3232

Website: www.liverdoctor.com
Website: www.sandracabot.com

© Sandra Cabot MD, 2015
ISBN 978-1-936609-24-6

HEA039090	HEALTH & FITNESS / Diseases / Immune & Autoimmune
HEA039010	HEALTH & FITNESS / Diseases / Gastrointestinal
HEA048000	HEALTH & FITNESS / Diet & Nutrition / General

Contents

Contents 3

Foreword 5

    How can gluten make us overweight? 6

Gluten Intolerance a hidden factor in illness 9

    How common is gluten intolerance? 12

    What are the clues that you may be gluten intolerant? 13

    What are the symptoms of gluten intolerance? 20

Diagnosis of Gluten Intolerance 21

    Gluten Elimination diet 25

Tips to help you quit gluten 26

    Sources of Gluten in the diet 28

    Gluten Free Foods are: 31

    Supplementation in the treatment of Gluten Sensitivity: 36

Gluten Free Healthy Recipes 42

    BREAKFASTS 42

        Summer Porridge 42

        Quick filling healthy yogurt 43

        Quinoa Porridge 43

        Corn pancakes 44

        Blueberry Coconut Muffins 44

        Other breakfast ideas 46

    LUNCHES 46

        Black rice salad with carrot and butternut pumpkin 46

        Whole grain corn muffins 48

    DINNERS 49

        Mexican roast sweet potato 49

        Amaranth Casserole Recipe 49

        Mediterranean Spaghetti Bolognese 50

        Chicken and Vegetable Soup 51

        Mexican Style Vegetarian Beans 52

        Tuna and Potato Salad 53

        Grilled Sardines with Lemon 53

Nori Rolls 54

Makes approx 10 rolls 54

Summer Chicken Kebabs 55

Chicken Omelette 56

Thai Green Chicken Curry. 57

Apricot Fat-Free Chicken. 58

Fresh Fish with Ginger and Spring Onions 59

Fish Steaks with Tangy Topping 60

Quick Beef and Mushroom Casserole. 61

Spicy Beef with Pulses 61

DESSERTS AND SWEET TREATS. 63

Chia pudding 63

Chocolate and Date Balls 63

Lemon Cookies 64

Muesli Bars. 64

Chocolate and Date Squares. 65

Chocolate and Orange Pudding. 66

Coconut Bread 66

Lemon Cheesecake Bars. 67

Processed Gluten Free Foods. 69

New developments under way 70

Summary 73

Autoimmune problems can vary widely. 73

Gluten and inflammation. 79

Beneficial Fermented Foods for the Digestive Tract. 82

Fermented Vegetable Recipe. 85

Mauritian Cabbage Pickle 85

One to two week liver and bowel detox program. 87

How are allergies mediated in the body?. 91

References 93

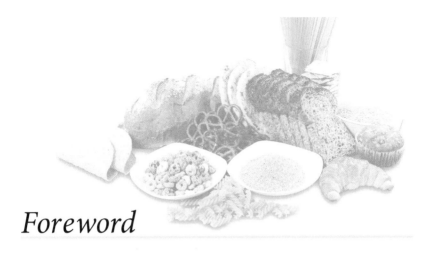

Foreword

Is it possible that gluten could cause such damage in your body that you become chronically unwell? Even if you are NOT a celiac, could gluten really make you very ill?

Many people have trouble believing this idea and I can understand why, as we have been educated to eat whole grains regularly for a balanced diet and good health. People think that grain based foods fill them up, stabilize blood sugar levels, provide fiber to help the bowels and keep weight down. I used to think that wholegrain wheat, rye and barley were healthy for everyone, but I don't anymore!

It is not just the amount of wheat that we eat but also the hidden components of wheat that drive weight gain and disease. This is not the wheat eaten by our forebears in the 19th century. It is vastly different so that it has become known as "FrankenWheat" or dwarf wheat. Dwarf wheat has been created via genetic manipulation and hybridization and is a short and stubby type of wheat. Dwarf wheat has much higher amounts of gluten and more chromosomes which code for all sorts of new odd proteins. Thus it brings us into unchartered waters.

In my practice I see a lot of chronically ill people, including many cancer patients, and most of them eat gluten. I have found that a significant percentage of these unwell people gradually restore their health when they give up gluten in their diet. They are not celiac but they are gluten intolerant – in other words the protein called gluten damages the cells in various parts of their body.

Gluten causes damage via the gut and the immune system where it causes inflammation. Immune cells are activated by gluten in the wrong way, so they become programmed to attack your cells. Gluten can cause very chronic, subtle and insidious damage that may never be recognized.

Gluten may cause gut inflammation causing the gut to become excessively permeable (this is known as leaky gut). This can cause your blood level of toxins to increase. Your intestines from the mouth to the anus can be damaged by gluten so that you do not absorb nutrients essential to health and longevity. Deficiencies of vitamin D, vitamin B 12, zinc, selenium and iron are common in gluten intolerant people. So if you have a healthy diet and take supplements you are unable to absorb them from your damaged or leaky gut. In other words you cannot get better and do not understand why.

How can gluten make us overweight?

We have been taught to think that excess fat and sugar makes us overweight, which as far as sugar is concerned is true. But can gluten alone make us overweight or stop us losing weight? You bet it can, I have seen it do this in hundreds of my patients.

Gluten containing foods are naturally high in carbohydrates and in many people they do not need to ingest this type of carbohydrate. They are much better off to get their carbohydrates from vegetables and gluten free grains – see page 31. But other non-gluten containing grains such as rice and corn are also high in carbohydrates – but they are not as fattening as gluten containing grains – very curious!

Why is this?

It is not the calories or the total amount of dietary carbohydrate that is the most important factor, but rather it is the type of molecules in the carbohydrates and how they affect your genes that trigger obesity. If you are gluten intolerant, gluten will turn on your fat genes.

Modern dwarf wheat may look like wheat, but it is different because:

- It contains a Super Drug that is super-addictive and makes you crave and overeat
- It contains a Super Starch called amylopectin A – this starch is super fattening

The Super Drug in gluten makes you hungry and potentially addicted to food. In the intestines the proteins in wheat are converted into shorter proteins called "polypeptides" or "exorphins". They are like the endorphins you get from narcotic pain killers. After they attach to the opioid receptors in the brain, you feel euphoric just like a heroin addict These wheat polypeptides are absorbed from the intestines into the bloodstream and get across the blood brain barrier quickly. They are called "gluteomorphins" after "gluten" and "morphine". Once in the brain they can cause addictive eating behavior and stimulate strong cravings for high carb foods and of course – more gluten!

In summary we can say that wheat is an addictive appetite stimulant!

Another way that gluten makes us overweight is that in many people it raises the blood levels of the hormone insulin. Higher insulin levels promote fat storage and hunger.

New dwarf wheat is very fattening – such that two slices of wholewheat bread now raise your blood sugar more than two tablespoons of table sugar!

In people with diabetes, both white and wholegrain bread raises blood sugar levels 70 to 120 mg/dl over starting levels. Thus the promoted idea that whole wheat grains are healthier than refined wheat grains has been turned on its head

The inflammation caused by gluten saps our energy so we become less inclined to exercise. Have you noticed that after eating a meal high in bread or pasta that you feel tired and slowed down? This is a sign that gluten is not good for you.

Many people try a gluten free diet for a few weeks only, and then seeing no huge improvement, they quit. I can understand this, as gluten foods can be just as addictive as high sugar foods – it is hard to resist and persist!

You need to know that it can take 12 months of a gluten free diet before all the gluten gets out of your body and before the gluten affected cells are fully repaired. This is disappointing, especially if you are a gluten lover. Thankfully there are many delicious gluten free alternatives that are available today, so you do not feel deprived. This book will give you many new ideas to satisfy your taste bud curiosities.

Gluten Intolerance
a hidden factor in illness

Gluten sensitivity is best described as a sensitivity or intolerance to the ingestion of the protein gluten, which is found in numerous different foods.

Gluten sensitivity or intolerance is also known as non-celiac gluten sensitivity (NCGS), as it occurs in people who do not have Celiac Disease. Yes that's correct - you can be intolerant to gluten even though you do NOT have Celiac Disease.

People with gluten sensitivity are unable to tolerate gluten in their diet and if they ingest it they may experience a vast array of symptoms. Gluten sensitivity is extremely common with an estimated 18 million Americans suffering from it. Many people may attribute their poor health to being run down or overstressed when in reality their underlying problem is actually associated with their diet. Recent studies have found that gluten sensitivity may be associated with our immune system. Gluten sensitivity is caused by abnormal immune responses. Gluten confuses our innate immune system, triggering it into an overreaction, even though it is not a direct threat to our health. This trigger creates a cascade of inflammation, not just in the gut, but throughout the body, causing excessive inflammation in different organs and tissues. The onset of gluten sensitivity can occur at any time throughout your life.

What is gluten?

Gluten is a protein which is found in many common foods in our diet. Gluten helps foods keep their structure, gives food an appetizing bouncy texture and helps bread rise and hold form. Gluten is widely used as an additive in foods which have low protein content, because it is so highly available and cheap. This means that gluten is often added to products without people knowing. Many products you use daily could have hidden gluten.

What is the Difference between Celiac Disease and Gluten Sensitivity?

It is important to distinguish the difference between these two conditions, even though they can be treated very similarly. Celiac Disease is a severe allergy to gluten, which manifests primarily as damage to the lining of the small intestine. People who suffer from Celiac Disease have abnormal immune systems, which produce antibodies against the antigen gluten and these antibodies attack gluten when it is ingested. These antibodies are not produced in people with gluten sensitivity who are not celiacs. The increased immune reaction which occurs with Celiac sufferers causes serious damage to the lining of the small intestine. In those people who are not celiacs, but nevertheless still suffer with Gluten Sensitivity, this damage to the small intestine does not occur. Therefore the diagnosis for Celiac Disease is vastly different to that of Gluten Sensitivity. People who show the symptoms of gluten reactivity may have

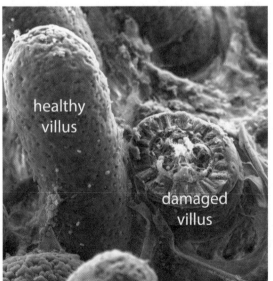

Small intestine villi. Coloured scanning electron micrograph of villi (brown) on the lining of the small intestine. Villi greatly increase the intestinal surface area for the absorption of nutrients from food. A broken villus is seen at lower right, revealing its internal structure. The villus epithelium (brown/blue in cross- section) contains enterocytes (light brown), which are involved in nutrient absorption. Scattered amongst these are goblet cells (blue), which secrete mucus onto the intestinal surface. Capillary blood vessels (red) within the villus transport digestive products to a nearby vein. Magnification: x190 at 6x6cm size. x300 at 4x5'

Photo Credit - Science Photo Library

to undergo numerous blood tests, stool tests, gastroscopies and biopsies to distinguish whether they have Celiac Disease or Gluten Sensitivity. Usually people who have negative test results for Celiac Disease still have Gluten sensitivity.

Normal Healthy Villi in the Small Intestine (left)   *Celiac Damaged Villi (right)*

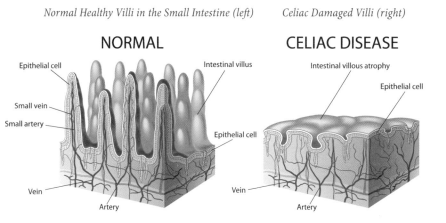

This diagram depicts the difference between a normal healthy small intestine, compared to that of a chronic celiac.

Villi are small finger like protrusions on the inner surface of the small intestine. Celiac sufferers have a greatly reduced surface area in their small intestine because of the damage caused to the villi. This reduces their ability to absorb most nutrients, resulting in severe nutrient deficiencies and malabsorption of fats and proteins. Understandably weight loss and poor health result. The inability to absorb fat from the intestines often results in diarrhea and fatty stools which float on the top of the water in the toilet after flushing the toilet.

How common is gluten intolerance?

Celiac disease prevalence has increased in the last few years. The true extent of gluten sensitivity and Celiac Disease in different ethnic populations is still in its very early years of study. The research that is currently available is only the tip of the iceberg; however it does shed some light on those races that are more susceptible to gluten reactivity.

Recent studies show that some ethnic groups have been found to have higher incidences of Celiac Disease. People from a Western European ancestry have a higher prevalence of gluten intolerance. Celiac Disease is more predominant in those from a Caucasian background, particularly from Celtic heritage.

There are some races that have very low prevalence of Celiac Disease. Celiac Disease is not commonly reported in ethnic populations in Africa, the Caribbean, China and Japan. However it is important to remember that these statistics may be inconsistent because of a lack of gluten containing foods in the local diet. This would mean that Celiac Disease sufferers would not show symptoms while eating their normal low gluten or gluten free diet. The quality and availability of medical resources in these countries might also mean that people are not getting diagnosed, even though they may suffer from gluten reactivity.

In Australia Celiac Disease affects 1 in 70 people. However a large proportion of people (80%) who have Celiac Disease are currently undiagnosed. This figure also doesn't take into account people who are gluten sensitive. Food intolerance incidences are also on the rise, with 1 in 25 people having food intolerance. In 2013 Dr Jason Tye-Din of The Walter and Eliza Hall Institute published new data showing the prevalence of Celiac Disease in Australia is much higher than previously estimated – it is now thought that around 340,000 Australians have Celiac Disease. Celiac disease is one of the most under diagnosed conditions in

Australia and the USA. It is estimated to affect 1 in 80 men and 1 in 60 women.

It is very important to think of Celiac Disease and to test for it in people who are unwell with no obvious cause. This is because if it remains undiagnosed and thus untreated, it can result in osteoporosis, impaired fertility, autoimmune disease and some types of cancer such as bowel cancer and lymphoma.

Those who are relatives of people with Celiac Disease have a huge 1 in 22 chance of becoming Celiac, with second degree relatives having a 1 in 39 chance. Women are more commonly diagnosed with Celiac Disease or gluten intolerance than are men.

What are the clues that you may be gluten intolerant?

There are many clues which can help you find out if you are gluten intolerant. Because gluten has the ability to cause inflammation throughout the whole body, your symptoms may not only be associated with your digestion and/or bowel function.

Here is a list of some key risk factors which may predispose you to Gluten Sensitivity:

Do you have inflammatory bowel disease such as Crohn's Disease or Ulcerative Colitis?

Both these diseases can be aggravated by Gluten Sensitivity. Having a family history of Celiac Disease, Ulcerative Colitis and/or Crohn's Disease can also predispose you to Gluten Sensitivity.

Do you have unexplained bowel problems for which your doctor can find no cause?

Symptoms such as reflux, indigestion, heartburn, irritable bowel syndrome, constipation, diarrhea, abdominal bloating and anal irritation can be a sign of gluten intolerance. Because Gluten Sensitivity can have such vague symptoms, and is so difficult to diagnose, it can sometimes go untreated for years.

Do you have rheumatoid, psoriatic or other types of inflammatory arthritis?

Sometimes joint inflammation can be triggered by food intolerances, especially gluten sensitivity. In fact all autoimmune conditions can be exacerbated by Gluten Sensitivity. Often people who have suffered from chronic joint inflammation really benefit from introducing a low inflammation, gluten free diet.

Do you have recurrent inflammatory skin problems?

Chronic inflammatory skin problems such as eczema, psoriasis or dermatitis are commonly found in people with hidden Gluten Sensitivity. The skin is our body's largest organ and a main organ of toxin elimination, so you can imagine it would be one of the first places we would notice an inflammatory reaction. It is also important to check cosmetic products, as they often have gluten added to them as a binder and you may experience contact dermatitis from this.

Dermatitis herpetiformis is a skin disease that is caused by gluten in the body. So when you take gluten out of the body, miraculously, for many people, the skin disease goes away. Dermatitis herpetiformis is a skin disease that is extremely itchy with blisters all over the body: on the back, on the scalp, even on the face, on the chest, on the arms. For some people even removing the gluten isn't enough to get rid of the skin disease completely, and they require an internal medication called colchicine. Colchicine and a gluten-free diet control the dermatitis herpetiformis. They also require supplements of zinc and selenium. The patient then has no itching, the skin bumps and blisters go away and the skin is totally clear.

Do you have unexplained deficiencies of minerals (especially zinc, iron and selenium) and/or vitamin D or vitamin B 12?

When people suffer from Gluten Sensitivity it often affects their ability to absorb nutrients from their small intestine, even though they are not technically a celiac person. If you have had chronic anemia due to unexplained low iron levels, you are probably gluten intolerant. Long standing low levels of zinc are often due to undiagnosed gluten sensitivity and will manifest as white spots in the nails, slow healing and a weakened immune system. Low levels of selenium are another common manifestation of gluten intolerance and will manifest as a weakened immune system. Low levels of zinc and/or selenium often manifest as mouth ulcers and frequent viral infections. Gluten intolerance can lead to very low levels of vitamin D in your body which will manifest as premature osteoporosis. If gluten causes inflammation in your stomach or the part of your bowel known as the ileum, this can result in low levels of vitamin B 12 in your body which manifests as anemia or poor mental health. Yes these deficiencies are often a sign that you are not absorbing nutrients efficiently because of gluten sensitivity.

Do you get recurrent infections and/or suffer from poor immune function?

When people have long standing chronic inflammation they require higher amounts of specific nutrients in their diet. Because Gluten Intolerant people often have multiple nutrient deficiencies and they are unable to absorb these vital nutrients from their diet their immune system is unable to recover. Poor immune function can lead to an increase in infections (such as influenza, sinusitis, bronchitis, candida and athletes foot) and also an increased risk of inflammation and cancer.

Do you have gastrointestinal problems?

Problems with digestion and bowel function are probably the most common manifestation of gluten insensitivity. Flatulence, abdominal pain and bloating may occur due to excess fermentation of gluten in the gut. This can also lead to foul smelling bowel motions, along with intermittent diarrhea or constipation which can be misdiagnosed as irritable bowel syndrome. Colonoscopy and gastroscopy and other tests may not show any definite abnormalities and so the true cause of gluten sensitivity is missed just because the patient is not a celiac.

Do you have excessive fatigue?

There is a strong link between Gluten Sensitivity and fatigue. Long term inflammation uses up your reserves of energy and uses greater amounts of essential nutrients needed for energy production. Unfortunately the hidden gluten intolerance makes it impossible for you to absorb these nutrients even though you may have a reasonable diet and take supplements.

Do you have mental fogginess and reduced cognitive ability?

The inflammation caused by Gluten Sensitivity does not stop at joints and skin. It can cause inflammation in the brain which damages neurones. Dr Perlmutter's excellent book titled **Grain Brain** explains the relationship between chronic brain inflammation and the development of neurodegenerative disorders such as dementia, Parkinson's disease and multiple sclerosis amongst others. Gluten intolerance can even damage a part of the brain known as the cerebellum and this can cause a gross disturbance of balance and movement (ataxia). This auto-immune ataxia disappears after gluten is removed from the diet. Gluten sensitivity can even aggravate headaches, sinusitis, abnormal movements and nerve pain.

Do you have joint and/or muscle pain or skin inflammation?

Unexplained inflammatory skin conditions and joint and muscle pain can often be caused by or exacerbated by gluten intolerance. Gluten triggers the immune system to start an inflammatory cascade in the connective tissues and skin, which can cause pain and even swelling in tissues in and around joints and ligaments. Nutrient malabsorption, particularly of magnesium, can trigger muscular cramps.

Do you have unexplained weight loss or weight gain?

Gut motility determines the time it takes for food to make its way through the gut and into the toilet bowl. When people suffer from food intolerances this can either become increased (meaning the transit time of food becomes faster) or decreased (meaning the transit time of food becomes too long). Gut motility can greatly affect weight loss and weight gain. Some nutrients which are essential to metabolism can also become deficient, leading to slower metabolism and weight gain. In celiac patients the severe malabsorption of fat, protein and carbohydrates causes weight loss but lesser degrees of gut damage from gluten that do not qualify for Celiac Disease, can also lead to some degree of malabsorption of macro-nutrients resulting in weight loss. In other people with gluten intolerance weight gain may occur because gluten makes them insulin resistant so their insulin levels rise. Insulin is a fat storing hormone and so they gain unwanted weight. Many type 2 diabetics have much better control of blood sugar levels when they follow a gluten free diet.

Do you have recurrent or persistent mouth ulcers?

Mouth ulcers are commonly associated with food intolerances and nutritional deficiencies. Recurrent mouth ulcers are often associated with Gluten Intolerance in particular. The deficiencies of zinc, selenium and vitamin D, which are prevalent in gluten intolerant people, make it hard for the ulcers to heal.

It's important to remember that not all people who have gluten sensitivity suffer from all of these symptoms and the symptoms can vary a lot in type and severity. This varied presentation makes it difficult for people who have gluten sensitivity to actually get diagnosed. Those who get diagnosed are just the tip of the iceberg.

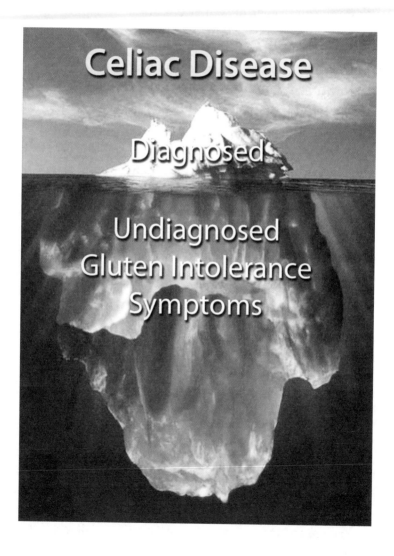

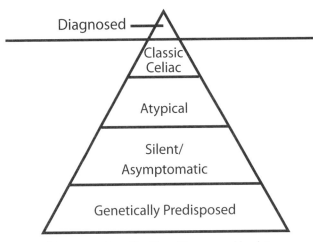

The presentation of health problems caused by gluten

This is because medical doctors are trained to recognize a definitive diagnosis of gluten intolerance only in patients with the classic criteria of Celiac Disease. The doctor will usually tell the patient "well you do not have Celiac Disease and thus you are not gluten intolerant". This is wrong and the patient remains unwell often for the rest of their life and especially as they get older or become stressed. Gluten intolerant people often do not handle vaccinations very well and eventually over vaccination can precipitate an autoimmune disease in such people – alas the connection with gluten intolerance is never recognized.

Many people with Gluten Sensitivity are asymptomatic, meaning they have no distinguishable symptoms. They may just have low energy, weight excess, grumbling arthritis or chronic skin conditions, which they do not directly relate to their diet. Some people may show no symptoms at all, but still react to gluten at a cellular level, which can cause chronic health conditions in the future. Some people are just genetic carriers of the susceptibility to gluten induced inflammation, and if they do not have any triggers, such as over vaccination, too many antibiotics or severe stress, they do not manifest the inflammation as a disease or significant symptoms.

What are the symptoms of gluten intolerance?

The symptoms associated with Gluten Sensitivity are wide and varied. People can suffer from all, or only some of these symptoms. Gluten intolerance can cause very vague and annoying symptoms or can eventually result in the manifestation of or aggravation of debilitating diseases.

Gluten Sensitivity often goes undiagnosed or mistreated for many years, if not for life, but it is important to start treating it sooner rather than later.

Long term undiagnosed Gluten Sensitivity can be very dangerous and can even result in a much higher risk of cancer. This is because of the long term inflammation and nutritional deficiencies caused by it.

See page 73 for more detailed information of symptoms and signs of non celiac gluten sensitivity (NCGS).

Diagnosis
of Gluten Intolerance

Blood Testing

Unfortunately Gluten Sensitivity is not always able to be accurately diagnosed or discovered in normal conventional blood tests. However blood tests play an important role in ruling out other serious bowel diseases like Celiac Disease. The antibodies which are produced in Celiac Disease are easily picked up in blood tests such as Celiac Disease Serology. There is a blood test available to detect abnormal sensitivity to gluten. It is called an antigliaden antibody test. This test is more accurate in children than in adults although it can give false results - either false positives or false negatives.

Celiac Disease Serology tests consist of-

Endomysial antibody .... negative or positive

Tissue Transglutaminase IgA .... negative is less than 15 U/mL

Tissue Transglutaminase IgG .... negative is less than 15 U/mL

Deamidated Gliadin IgA .... negative is less than 15 U/mL

Deamidated Gliadin IgG .... negative is less than 15 U/mL

Total Serum IgA .... negative is less than 3.10 g/L

Interpretation of these antibody tests

- In a person eating wheat, the presence of one positive antibody may occur without Celiac Disease being present. Multiple positive antibodies strongly predict Celiac Disease, which can be confirmed by biopsy of the small intestinal lining via endoscopy. In monitoring Celiac Disease, IgA antibodies may become negative after 6 to 9 months, while IgG antibodies take longer to disappear (up to 12 months). This confirms the fact that it takes around 12 months for the damaging effects of gluten allergy to get out of your body and thus for your health to improve. It also confirms the need to follow a strict gluten free diet.

- It is possible to have more in-depth tests for gluten intolerance and also for intolerance to other foods (especially grains) that cross react with gluten. These tests are expensive but some people will still choose to have them especially if they remain unwell after following a gluten free diet for 12 months. For more information see www.cyrexlabs.com/CyrexTestsArrays

- RAST testing tests for gluten allergy. A positive test indicates gluten allergy, however you can have negative RAST tests and still be classified as gluten sensitive.

- Other blood tests which are helpful in the diagnosis of Gluten Sensitivity include; serum carotene, vitamin A, vitamin D, B12, zinc, selenium, iron studies and folate. In most people with gluten intolerance the levels of these nutrients will be abnormally low.

Genetic test

The HLA-DQ genotype test is a relatively new blood test which can check if you have the genetic pattern that predisposes you to gluten intolerance or Celiac Disease. People are born with a genetic predisposition to developing Celiac Disease. They inherit a particular genetic make-up (HLA –DQ type), with the genes HLA-DQ2 and HLA-DQ8 being identified as the 'Celiac genes'. More than 95% of persons with Celiac Disease have either the HLA-DQ2 or HLA-DQ8 genetic pattern, but not all of them will get Celiac Disease; however they are more likely to have Non Celiac Gluten Sensitivity (NCGS).

If you are found to have this genetic make-up then you may be a carrier of Celiac Disease, or you could have undiagnosed Non Celiac Gluten Sensitivity (NCGS). In many cases, gluten intolerance or even Celiac Disease will not have been diagnosed in previous family generations. However, a first-degree relative (brother, sister, parent or child) of a person with Celiac Disease has about a 10 per cent chance of also having the condition. Even if you do NOT have the HLADQ 2 and HLADQ 8 genetic pattern that is associated with Celiac Disease you may still be gluten sensitive, so this blood test is just a guide. If you are negative for this test you may still benefit from a gluten free diet which could alleviate your symptoms.

Skin prick testing

- Skin prick testing involves pricking the skin with small amounts of allergens, to see if there is any reaction, such as swelling and redness.

- The amount the skin prick swells corresponds with the degree of the allergy.

- There are some limitations to skin prick testing. This testing only works on certain types of allergies, specifically IgE mediated allergies. This means that if an allergy is not an IgE mediated allergy it will not show a positive result. See page 91 for more information on how food allergies are mediated

Stool sample tests

Incompletely digested foods may be found in stool sample tests due to increased gut motility and malabsorption. This can be caused by food intolerances such as gluten. The feces can be tested for blood and bacteria and parasites to exclude other causes of bowel diseases. Specialised tests known as a "Complete Diagnostic Stool Analysis" (CDSA) can be done by doctors and naturopaths interested in nutritional medicine.

The CDSA is divided into panel A and panel B.

Panel A assesses the overall appearance of your bowel actions (stools), as well as checking them for blood cells and fat globules. It also measures the stools for markers of food digestion and absorption, such as triglyceride fats, chymotrypsin enzyme, meat fibers, vegetable cells and fibers, acid-base balance, and short chain fatty acids such as valerate and iso-butyrate, long chain fatty acids, cholesterol and total fecal fat. Panel A will give your doctor a very good evaluation of your ability to digest and absorb a wide range of food groups. This is important because even though you may have an excellent diet, you may not be able to extract the vital nutrients from your food if your liver, gallbladder, pancreas, stomach or intestines are malfunctioning.

Panel B assesses the types and amounts of microorganisms in your gut. This is done using microscopy and cultures to look for parasites, bacteria and fungi.

Gluten Elimination diet

- The best way to test if you are gluten intolerant is to eliminate ALL gluten containing foods from your diet for 3 to 6 months and observe the difference in your health and your bowel function. It is important to remove ALL gluten, so make sure you check the labels of everything you eat. Gluten is a thickening agent and is constantly added to processed foods such as; salad dressings, sauces, stock and soup mixes, and even to certain brands of vitamins or medications.

- If you fail to remove ALL the gluten from your diet, your immune system will still be reacting to small particles of gluten leaving you with low grade systemic inflammation throughout your body. This will mean that your symptoms will not completely resolve.

- After this period, eat gluten again and see how you feel. This is called "challenge testing". If you feel unwell or bad in any way after eating gluten, then you should stay off gluten permanently. Remember that it may not only be your bowel movements that are affected. Check your skin tone, general mood, energy levels and even quality of sleep.

Tips to help you quit gluten

Gluten can be addictive and renowned neurologist Dr Perlmutter says that gluten can produce a type of excitatory high feeling when it over-stimulates neurones. Thus some people find it really hard to quit gluten. Also they think that if they are not a celiac sufferer, and this myth is often reinforced by their doctor, that they do not really need to eliminate ALL gluten from their diet – this is false. We admit it can be as hard as quitting sugar, nicotine or alcohol, but it is worth it for your health

- Changing your diet to one without gluten seems quite difficult at first but with a little practise it gets a lot easier. You will be rewarded with feelings of vitality and wellbeing once you've accomplished a complete abstinence from gluten. It may take up to 12 months to completely heal the damage that gluten has caused in your body, so be patient. Yes that's right – it can take up to 12 months for gluten to get out of your body!

- If you are attempting to lose weight through gluten free dieting, the first thing to remember is that many processed packaged GLUTEN FREE foods are still high in other gluten free carbohydrates, sugar, preservatives and vegetable oils (trans-fats). So while trying to lose weight you need to go on a low carbohydrate eating plan and will need to minimize things like pasta, bread, cereals, biscuits and cakes, even if they are gluten free. These foods are fairly nutrient poor and calorie rich. These are referred to as empty foods.

- Choose protein that is fresh and unprocessed (such as lean red meat, chicken, eggs or seafood, plain yogurt, unprocessed cheeses) and a delicious fresh salad for dinner without worrying about hidden gluten. Remember Dr Cabot's Synd X Slimming Protein Powder and QuickLoss Meal Replacement do not contain any gluten so you can safely enjoy your protein/meal replacement shakes while trying to lose weight safely. Processed meats, such as devon and sausages often contain hidden gluten. Make your own sauces or salad dressings from cold pressed olive oil, lime, lemon or apple cider vinegar, as bottled salad dressings, as well as many gravies, contain gluten. Alternatively, find a reliable source of healthy low sugar gluten free dressings and sauces.

- Good gluten free snacks include raw seeds and nuts, canned fish, avocado, cheese, fruit, plain unsweetened yogurt or high protein, low carb gluten free snack bars . . . Too easy!

Reminder

Whether you test positive to gluten intolerance or not you may find a large improvement in your general health if you follow a gluten free diet. It can take up to 6 to 12 months before you can really judge the benefit, so you need to be strict and patient. Many tests used to assess Gluten Sensitivity are not completely accurate and this is why a gluten elimination diet may be the best way to discover if you are gluten intolerant.

Sources of Gluten in the diet

Gluten is found in many foods. Naturally gluten is found in the grains wheat, barley, rye and spelt. Some types of oats also contain gluten so it is best to avoid oats.

The type of gluten found within each of these grains differs; therefore some people are able to eat some and not others. But while you are testing a completely gluten free diet please avoid them all. These grains and their flours and other derivative products are found in breads, cereals, crackers, biscuits, muffins, cakes, pizza, pastry and pasta.

Grains to avoid are:

Wheat

Wheat contains the highest amount of gluten out of all the gluten containing grains, indeed up to 80%. Although wheat naturally has high gluten levels it has recently increased further due to plant genetic modifications. Selective breeding has greatly modified wheat over the last 100 years to produce higher yields, improve disease resistance and create better bread-making characteristics. This particular type of wheat is often found in everyday supermarket foods and may be associated with the increased incidence of gluten intolerance we see today.

Other examples of wheat varieties include faro, spelt, kamut and

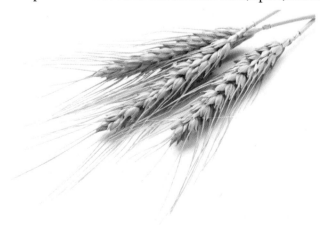

durum. However these grains usually have not been selectively bred and therefore contain their natural amount of gluten, rather than artificially raised levels. However avoid them on a gluten free diet.

Oats

It is believed that some types of oats contain small amounts of gluten, and as well many people react to oats due to cross-contamination with gluten, as many factories that process oats, also process wheat grain. Therefore it is important to source gluten free oats when using them during a gluten free diet, or even better avoid oats completely.

Barley

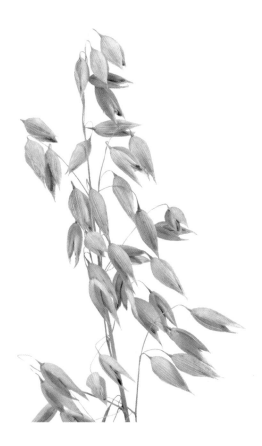

Barley contains smaller amounts of gluten compared to wheat therefore some people are able to digest it. However if you are following a completely gluten free diet, then you will need to eliminate all barley products, as people can react to even the smallest amounts of gluten.

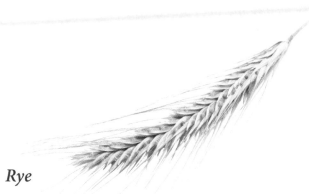

Rye

Rye is one of the most recently domesticated crops; this means that it has been bred selectively for fewer years than wheat has and still contains a similar nutrient content as when it was grown from the wild. Avoid rye whilst on a gluten free diet.

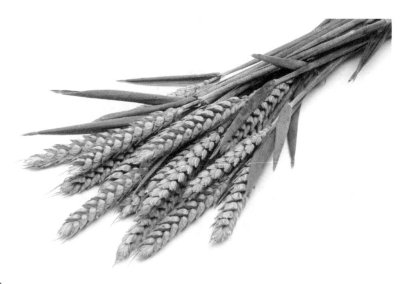

Gluten Free Foods are:

After reading which grains you need to eliminate from your diet, you may be thinking there is nothing left to eat. But hang on you will not go hungry! There are many other gluten free grains which can replace those containing gluten such as rice, tapioca, arrowroot, maize, millet, sago, buckwheat, amaranth and quinoa. Nuts, legumes (lentils, beans and chickpeas) and seeds are also gluten free.

Amaranth

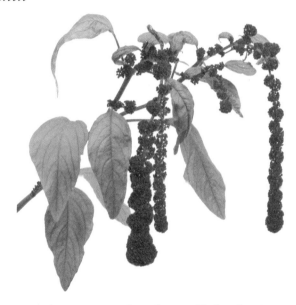

Amaranth was the grain used traditionally by the Aztec Indians of North America. Amaranth is now becoming a popular again amongst health conscious people. It is very high in protein and is a good source of complex carbohydrates. Amaranth is gluten free and can be used as a substitute for wheat in those with Gluten Sensitivity. It needs to be pre-soaked and cooked on a low heat to aid in digestion. It is excellent for casseroles and stews. It can also be bought as a puffed grain and used for a healthy breakfast muesli.

Buckwheat

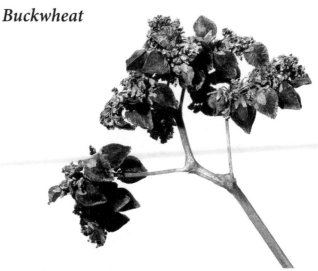

Even though buckwheat has wheat in its name, it is not a wheat grain. Buckwheat is completely gluten free and is a fantastic source of essential nutrients, fiber and energy. Buckwheat is incredibly high in protein and contains excellent supplies of zinc, copper and manganese. Buckwheat can be eaten raw, sprouted, or it can be cooked up like porridge.

Corn

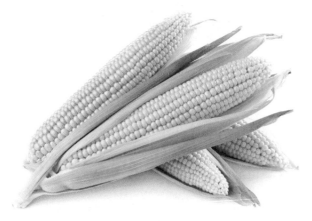

Corn and cornmeal can be eaten while abstaining from gluten. It is excellent for making corn breads and polenta. Popped corn makes a tasty snack.

Millet

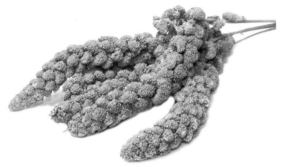

Millet naturally contains no gluten and can be consumed by those with Celiac Disease and gluten sensitivity; however millet sometimes becomes contaminated with wheat and other sources of gluten during harvesting, storage and processing of mixed crops. Millet can be puffed, boiled and eaten whole, or ground into flour.

Quinoa

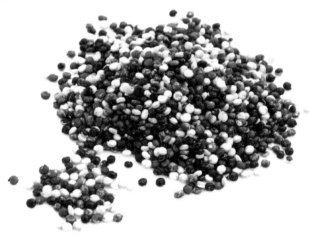

Quinoa is another ancient grain and was traditionally used by the Incas. It is high in protein and can be used as a substitute for wheat in many dishes. Quinoa is gluten free and is tolerated well by those with Gluten Sensitivity. It is also good for those with intolerance to dairy products because it is very high in calcium, helping to supplement the diet which often lacks calcium.

Rice

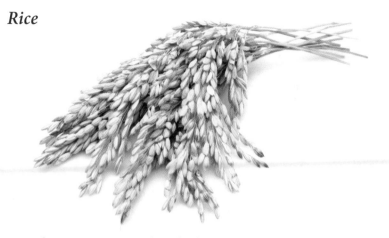

Rice does contain starch, which gives it a sticky consistency but it does not contain gluten proteins. Thankfully rice is completely gluten free. When choosing rice try to choose brown grains or if you prefer white rice, choose basmati rice, which has a lower glycemic index than other white rice, so will make you feel fuller for longer. Also keep an eye out for alternative types of rice, such as black rice, coral rice and wild rice. These types of rice are excellent sources of fiber, nutrients and minerals.

Sorghum

Sorghum is an ancient grain which originates from Africa. Sorghum is one of the only grains with an edible hull, making it incredibly nutritious and high in fiber. It is completely gluten free and makes a great replacement for wheat flour.

Teff

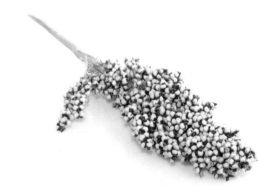

Teff is a very small grain often used in making flat breads after being fermented. It is incredibly nutritious with excellent amounts of calcium, magnesium and vitamin C. You can also eat teff whole by cooking 1 cup of teff to 3 cups of water for 20 minutes.

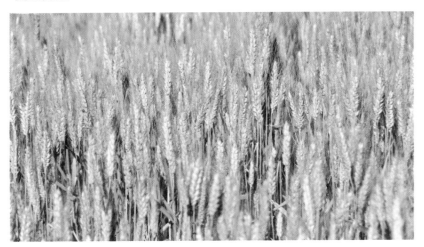

Other gluten-free foods:

Naturally poultry, meat, seafood, eggs, dairy products, nuts, seeds and legumes, vegetables and fruits are all gluten free.

There are many gluten free products available today and mandatory correct labeling has made it much easier to find gluten free foods. But always read the labels very carefully on any product first before purchasing. Gluten-free (GF) bread, GF pasta, GF biscuits, GF crackers, GF muesli and GF flour are easily available at most supermarkets and health stores. They are usually made from such things as potato, hemp seeds, chick peas, peas, soy and rice. Often replacement ingredients are added to products to give them a glutinous texture. These include xanthan gum, potato starch, agar agar and guar gum. These are all gluten free and can be freely used during gluten free dieting.

There are numerous restaurants now that specialize in gluten free meals. Some pizza houses make gluten free pizzas if you request it. However if you have Celiac Disease then you may choose not to have the pizza where regular gluten pizzas are made, as there could be cross contamination of gluten particles from the pizza oven or the utensils.

Supplementation in the treatment of Gluten Sensitivity:

There are specific supplements which can help heal the gut and reduce the symptoms associated with Gluten Sensitivity. These supplements can gradually restore normal levels of vital nutrients in the body provided the diet remains gluten free to enable the gut lining to repair.

Using these supplements along with implementing a strict gluten free diet can completely eliminate specific health complaints associated with Gluten Sensitivity.

L-Glutamine

If your diagnosis of Celiac Disease was delayed until later in life, the long term ingestion of gluten may have caused damage to your small and/or large intestine and this may take several years to completely repair. To speed up the repair of your gut lining I recommend glutamine powder because glutamine is used by the cells lining the gut as a fuel for energy and also to renew new healthy intestinal cells. Glutamine powder is taken in a dose of 2 to 5 grams (1/2 to one teaspoon) once or twice daily in sugar free milk (such as dairy, coconut, rice or almond milk). Use a cool beverage as glutamine is degraded by heat. Gluten can also be added to smoothies

Vitamin D

Vitamin D is a fat soluble vitamin that requires fat in the diet and a healthy gut to be absorbed in adequate amounts. Vitamin D is not really a vitamin and has now been correctly classified as a hormone that regulates hundreds of our genes to keep our immune system healthy. It is also different from all other nutrients because it is mostly made in our body from UVB light produced by the sun. Most gluten intolerant people are very low in vitamin D and this makes their inflammation much worse. Vitamin D deficiency also leads to premature or severe osteoporosis and this is common in people with undiagnosed gluten intolerance.

It is vitally important to ask your doctor to check your blood level of vitamin D. The correct blood test is called 25(OH) D, also called 25-hydroxyvitamin D3.

The most important factor is your vitamin D serum level. It doesn't matter how much time you spend in the sun, or how much vitamin D3 you take: if your serum level is low, then you're at an increased risk of cancer and osteoporosis. The only way to know your serum level is to have a blood test. It's recommended you check your level every three to six months, because it takes at least three months for it to stabilize after a change in sun exposure or supplement dose.

Vitamin D can be measured in two different units of measurement and in the USA the units used are ng/mL. In Australia and Canada the units of measurement are nmol/L.

The normal ranges of vitamin D for blood tests reported by different laboratories and countries vary significantly and you will be surprised by the large range between lower normal and upper normal – see table below

Lower Limit Vitamin D	Upper Limit Vitamin D
75 nmol/L	200nmol/L
30 ng/mL	100ng/mL

You don't want to be average here; you want to have levels of vitamin D that optimize your immune system and the optimal levels of vitamin D are higher than the average levels.

I recommend you take enough supplements of vitamin D 3 and/ or get enough sunshine to keep your serum vitamin D levels around 150 to 200nmol/L or 70 to 100ng/mL. Vitamin D 3 supplements are not expensive. The best way to optimize your vitamin D level is through sun exposure, but for some people this is not practical or possible, especially during the winter months. As a very general guide, you need to expose 40 percent of your entire skin to the sun for 20 minutes between the hours of 10 am and 2 pm; this is when the sun is at its zenith. There appears to be no risk of vitamin D toxicity from ultraviolet B exposure.

If you're using an oral supplement, recent studies suggest adults need around 3000 to 8,000 IU's of oral vitamin D3 per day in order to get serum levels above 40 ng/ml. But this can vary a lot between individuals. Even the conservative Institute of Medicine has concluded that taking up to 10,000 IU per day poses no risk for adverse effects.

Excess vitamin D intake can cause elevated blood calcium levels; so don't overdose on it - it's not a case of the more the better. Get your blood level checked every 6 months to find the dose of vitamin D 3 that keeps you in the optimal levels.

Iron supplements

Iron supplements will be needed in gluten intolerant people who are low in iron. People with severe iron deficiency will show signs of anemia in their blood count and they will usually be very tired. If oral iron supplements do not work and you remain low in iron after several months of oral iron supplements, you should have a course of iron injections. The best brand of iron injections is called Ferinject. Iron injections can be astoundingly invigorating for those with chronic malabsorption of iron due to gluten induced gut damage.

Blood tests for iron should measure serum iron levels and

ferritin levels. Your iron levels can be compared to your financial situation – serum iron levels shows the ready cash you have whereas ferritin levels show the amount of money you have stored in your bank accounts. Low ferritin levels mean you are very low in iron and probably have been for a long time.

Zinc supplements

Blood zinc levels should be checked but may not be a true reflection of chronically low zinc, so a zinc supplement is worthwhile if gluten intolerance has weakened your immune system. I recommend a zinc supplement in a dose of 25mg daily with food.

Selenium supplements

Selenium deficiency is very common in gluten intolerant people and blood tests for selenium levels do not show your real total body selenium levels. You may have selenium blood levels within the normal range but still be deficient in this vital mineral. This is because gluten intolerance reduces the absorption of selenium, as well as zinc absorption, plus gluten intolerant people have higher requirements for selenium. Selenium is needed by your immune system to fight inflammation, infections and cancer, so you do not want to be low in selenium. Selenium deficiency is associated with a higher risk of many types of cancer such as thyroid, breast, skin and bowel cancer. Gluten intolerant people have a higher risk of bowel cancer and lymphoma and selenium supplementation can reduce this risk. I recommend 200mcg of a selenium supplement daily. See www.seleniumresearch.com

Vitamin B 12 supplements

Blood levels of Vitamin B 12 should be checked, as gluten intolerance can cause gastritis and bowel inflammation, which can lead to malabsorption of vitamin B 12 from foods. Vitamin B 12 deficiency can be due to the autoimmune condition of pernicious anemia and this means that oral vitamin B 12 cannot be absorbed from foods or supplements. In such cases injections of vitamin B 12 should be given every 6 weeks. Even if you do not have pernicious anemia, if your blood vitamin B 12 levels are low, you should take B 12 supplements.

Make sure you supplement with good quality supplements and if you need to, get guidance from a qualified naturopath, dietitian or nutritionist as to which nutrients you are lacking. You may email my Health Advisory Service from our websites www.liverdoctor.com or www.drsandracabotclinics.com.au

Digestive enzymes

Taking digestive enzymes with meals will help the digestion and absorption of carbohydrates, protein and fats from foods.

Probiotics

- The gut has a complicated flora of bacteria growing within it which is often compromised in people with food sensitivities. Not only do these bacteria help with the digestion of carbohydrates, they are also essential to our immunity. Different probiotic bacteria have been found to be beneficial in treating symptoms commonly associated with gluten sensitivity.

These probiotics include:

- Lactobacillus rhamnosus – is often used in the treatment of eczema
- Lactobacillus plantarum – used in the treatment of IBS symptoms
- Saccharomyces bourlardii – helps to restore healthy gut flora

Omega 3 fatty acids

Omega 3 fatty acids reduce inflammation and improve gut and immune health and many gluten intolerant people are deficient in these essential fats. A deficiency results in dry itchy skin and dry lifeless hair. It is important to boost the intake of omega 3 essential fatty acids by eating oily fish, chia seeds, hemp seeds, ground flaxseeds and walnuts. Avocados and coconut oil or coconut milk also boost the amount of healthy fats needed to reduce inflammation. If you are particularly affected by arthritis or joint pain you may find fish oil supplementation beneficial.

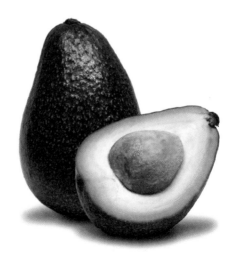

Gluten Free Healthy Recipes

BREAKFASTS

Summer Porridge

Ingredients

1 cup	cooked brown rice
1 tbsp	chia seeds
1 tbsp	raw buckwheat
1 tbsp	hemp seeds
1 tbsp	natural yogurt
2 tbsp	ground flaxseeds
1	apple grated
½ cup	frozen or fresh berries

Method

Mix the chia, buckwheat and apple in a small bowl with ½ cup of water and leave to soak overnight in the fridge. If you are using frozen berries then put the amount you want on top of the mixture. In the morning add cooked rice, hemp seeds, yogurt and ground flaxseeds.

Quick filling healthy yogurt

Ingredients

6 tbsp	full fat Greek yogurt
2 tbsp	LSA
2 tbsp	hemp seeds
1 tbsp	chia seeds (soak for 5 minutes)
2	passion fruit or 1 banana or other fruit of choice

Method

Mix all ingredients together and serve. This is a wonderful breakfast for those with constipation.

Quinoa Porridge

Ingredients

250g	quinoa grains
½ stick	cinnamon
125mL	fresh apple juice (not from concentrate, no added sugar) or juice yourself
325mL	water

Method

Place the quinoa, cinnamon, apple juice and 325mL water in a medium sized saucepan and bring to the boil. Lower the heat and simmer for 7-10 minutes, until the grains are translucent. Turn off the heat and allow to stand for 10 minutes. Enjoy!

Corn pancakes

Ingredients

3/4	cup gluten free medium cornmeal
1/2	cup tapioca flour
1/4	cup potato starch
2 tsp	Gluten Free baking powder
1/2 tsp	Himalayan sea salt
1/4 tsp	Xanthan gum
1 1/4 cups	unsweetened milk (almond or rice)
2 tbsp	coconut oil
1	egg, slightly beaten

Method

In a medium bowl, mix together the dry ingredients. Add the milk, oil and egg to the dry ingredients and whisk to incorporate until smooth. Prepare the pan by heating it on medium high heat and lightly oil it. Pour a ¼ cup of batter onto the prepared pan and cook until bubbles start to form, about 2 minutes. Flip the pancakes and cook the other side until the pancake is cooked through. Serve with your favorite toppings such as fresh fruit, hemp seeds or Greek yogurt.

Blueberry Coconut Muffins

Ingredients

8 oz	fresh or frozen blueberries
2	Tbsp coconut cream
3	Eggs, whole
2	Tbsp butter
2	Tbsp honey
¼	tsp sea salt

¼	tsp vanilla, organic, additive-free
¼	cup coconut flour
1/2	tsp baking soda

Method

Blend eggs, butter, coconut cream, honey, salt, and vanilla together.

Then combine coconut flour and baking powder and add to batter; make sure you smooth out all the lumps.

Wash and drain blueberries, dry thoroughly and add to batter.

Pour batter into muffin cups. Bake at 400 degrees F (205 C) for around 15 minutes. - *Makes 6 muffins*

GF Pancakes

Ingredients

4	eggs, whole
1/4 cup	GF flour (can choose coconut flour, hemp flour or rice flour)
1/4 tsp	vanilla extract
3 pinch	nutmeg
3 pinch	cinnamon
1 tablespoon	honey
1/4 cup	full fat dairy milk or coconut milk

Method

Mix all ingredients in a blender and let them sit for five minutes. Oil or grease up your pan and heat over medium heat. Pour about a 1/4 cup of batter for each pancake/crepe. Cook so that each side is brown before flipping it.

Other breakfast ideas

- Scrambled eggs with grilled tomatoes and GF bacon

- Poached eggs with GF bacon

- Hash browns with grilled vegetables

- Protein powder smoothie made with milk (coconut, dairy, rice or almond milk) and fruit

LUNCHES

Black rice salad with carrot and butternut pumpkin

Ingredients

3	*Cups black rice or wild rice*
½	*large butternut pumpkin*
2	*fresh beetroots*
½	*cup pepitas, toasted*
3	*spring onions, sliced*
2	*tbsp extra virgin olive oil*
1	*cup quinoa*
2	*tbsp red wine vinegar*
½	*bunch parsley*
¼	*cup lime juice*

Mint leaves to garnish

Method

Cook quinoa with 2 cups of boiling water until tender. In a separate saucepan place the black rice with 7 cups of boiling water, then lower heat and cook for 30-40mins with the lid on. Once both the quinoa and rice are cooked, rinse under cold water and set aside.

Dice the butternut pumpkin and beetroot into 2.5cm (1 inch)

cubes and place on a well oiled tray and bake for 30-40mins. While the vegetables are cooking toast the pepitas in a pan. Add the pumpkin, beetroot, spring onions, pepitas, quinoa and black rice into a large bowl and mix. Garnish with mint, parsley, red wine vinegar and lime juice.

Gluten-free Tabbouleh

Ingredients:

175g	*raw buckwheat*
6	*tbsp chopped mint*
12	*tbsp chopped parsley*
1	*large tomato, halved*
1	*cucumber, diced*
2	*onions, peeled and diced*
1	*tbsp virgin olive oil*
1	*tsp of dried mixed herbs*

Juice of 1 lemon

Sea salt and pepper to taste

Method

Rinse and drain the buckwheat. Bring a medium-sized pan of water to the boil, add the buckwheat and cook for 10 minutes until tender. Mix the mint, parsley, tomato, cucumber, onion, olive oil, lemon juice and dried mixed herbs together in a large bowl. Mix through the buckwheat and chill until required.

Whole grain corn muffins – makes 12

Ingredients

1 1/2 cups medium grind cornmeal

1 cup gluten free pastry flour

1 tbsp gluten free baking powder

2 tbsp evaporated cane juice

1/2 tsp sea salt

1 egg, lightly beaten

1 cup rice milk

1/4 cup refined coconut oil

Method:

Preheat oven to 180C. Grease a standard or mini muffin pan and set aside. Mix together the cornmeal, GF pastry flour, GF baking powder, cane juice and salt. Add the milk, egg and oil and blend until smooth, careful not to over mix. Spoon batter into the muffin tins about 3/4 full. Bake for about 20 minutes for the standard size and 12 minutes for the mini muffins. When done, tops of the muffins should spring back when tapped. These can be stored frozen. Serve with fresh salad or fresh fruit. Can be used for breakfast, lunch or a snack.

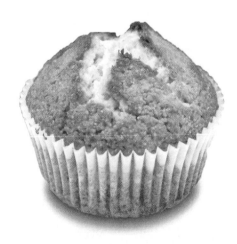

DINNERS

Mexican roast sweet potato

Ingredients

For each person

1	Whole sweet potato
2	tbsp gluten free vegetable stock
2	tbsp natural yogurt
¼	can unsweetened corn or equiv fresh corn scraped from cob

½ can mixed beans

Fresh coriander for garnish

Method

Preheat over to 200C. Place the sweet potato on a baking tray and roast for 45min. While the potato is roasting, heat the corn and mixed beans over a hotplate until warm. Once the sweet potato is soft in the center, remove from oven and slice in half. Pour the vegetable stock over the potato. Leave to cool for 5min and then add the corn and bean mix and top with natural yogurt and coriander.

Amaranth Casserole Recipe - Serves 4

Ingredients

1 cup	Amaranth, cooked
1 cup	Rice or millet, cooked
3 cloves	Garlic
1 cup	Carrots, sliced
1 cup	Cabbage, chopped
1	Zucchini, chopped
1 cup	Capsicum (bell pepper) chopped

1 cup	Fresh tomatoes, chopped
425g (15oz)	Whole tomatoes, tinned, chopped (keep juice)
4 tbsp	Olive Oil, cold pressed
3 tbsp	Fresh basil
2	Shallots, chopped
2	Brown onions, chopped

Method

Sauté olive oil with garlic, shallots and onions. Add all vegetables and sauté for 4 minutes.

- Add canned tomatoes and their juice, amaranth and rice (or millet).

- Simmer for 10 minutes and season to taste with sea salt, tamari, gluten free soy sauce or vegetable seasoning.

- Make sure the vegetables are still crisp and do not overcook.

Mediterranean Spaghetti Bolognese – Serves 4

Ingredients

2	tbsp olive oil
350g	pack lean beef or lamb mince
1	onion, peeled and diced
1	large carrot, peeled and grated
200g	mushrooms, sliced
100g	black olives
2 - 4	cloves garlic, chopped (optional)
1 tsp	dried mixed herbs or 2 tbsp fresh chopped herb
250ml	gluten free vegetable stock
400g	gluten free spaghetti
1	400g can chopped tomatoes or fresh tomatoes
2	tbsp gluten free tomato paste

Handful of rocket and salt and pepper, to season

Method

Heat the oil in a large frying pan and sauté onions and garlic until translucent. Add the mince and brown while breaking it up. Once cooked add the carrot into the pan and cook over heat, stirring frequently, for about 10 minutes, until soft. Add the mushrooms and fry for a few minutes more. Tip the tomatoes into the pan with the herbs, tomato paste and stock, then stir well to make a sauce. Season with salt and pepper, then cover and simmer for 12 minutes, until the vegetables are cooked and the mixture is saucy rather than wet.

Meanwhile, bring a large saucepan of salted water to the boil. Add the spaghetti and boil according to pack instructions until just tender. Drain the spaghetti and pile into four bowls. Spoon the sauce on top and garnish with black olives and rocket.

Chicken and Vegetable Soup - *Serves 6*

Ingredients

4	*Chicken drumsticks, free range or organic is best*
2 cups	*Carrots, chopped*
½ cup	*Parsley, chopped*
1 cup	*Swede, grated*
1 cup	*Parsnip, chopped*
1 cup	*Celery, chopped*
400g can	*Whole corn, including liquid or use fresh corn from cob*
1	*Large onion, chopped and browned in pan*

Method

Place all ingredients in a large pan and barely cover with water.

Bring to the boil and simmer for 1 hour until tender.

Remove chicken bones and leave the meat in the soup.

Season with pepper and sea salt to taste.

Suitable to freeze in serving portions.

Mexican Style Vegetarian Beans - *Serves 4 - 6*

Ingredients

	450g/16oz Red kidney beans, canned, drained or cooked
1 large	*Onion, chopped*
3 large	*Garlic cloves, chopped*
1 tbsp	*Cold pressed olive oil*
1 tbsp	*Tomato paste (more if desired)*
1 tsp	*Oregano, fresh*
1 tbsp	*Parsley, fresh chopped*
1 tbsp	*Basil, fresh chopped*
1 pinch	*Chilli powder and paprika (optional)*
	A little water
	Sea salt and cracked pepper to taste

Method

Brown onion and garlic in oil in large pan.

Add all other ingredients plus enough water to bind together.

Don't make it too moist, warm through.

Serve with rice, chopped tomatoes, sliced lettuce, alfalfa sprouts.

Mashed avocado may also be added if you desire.

Top with some chilled Greek yogurt.

Tuna and Potato Salad - *Serves 2 or more*

Ingredients

1/4 cup	Cold pressed olive oil
2 tbsp	Tamari (wheat free soy sauce)
1	Red salad onion, peeled and sliced finely
225g/8oz	Tuna
1/2	Iceberg lettuce, washed and torn up
1	Garlic clove, crushed
1	Lemon juiced
1	Lebanese cucumber, sliced lengthways
1 Punnett	Cherry tomatoes, washed
8 small	Tomatoes, chopped
4	Eggs, hard boiled and quartered
8 small	New potatoes, steamed, left to cool, then quartered

Method

Combine oil, tamari, lemon juice and some salt and set aside.

Put remaining ingredients into a large serving bowl and mix gently.

Pour dressing over salad and set aside for 5 mins before serving.

Grilled Sardines with Lemon - *Serves 4*

Ingredients

1kg/36oz	Sardines, fresh (filleted)

Marinade

6 tbsp	Cold pressed olive oil
2	Garlic cloves, finely chopped
1/2 cup	Lemon juice
4 tbsp	Coriander, chopped

Salt and black pepper to taste

Method

Brush the fish with oil and pour half the marinade on each side.

Brush with marinade each turn.

Serve with the remaining marinade poured over the top and a vegetable salad or a big green salad and Gluten free bread may be served on the side.

Nori Rolls

Makes approx 10 rolls

You will need a sushi mat for this recipe, which you can get from some supermarkets or an Asian grocery store. Try using different ingredients like prawns, tofu, tuna and salmon. Great for lunches, entrees and snacks.

Ingredients

5 sheets	Nori seaweed
1 med	Avocado
1 bunch	Garlic chives
2	Lebanese cucumbers
3 tbsp	LSA (linseeds, sunflower seeds and almonds – ground)
2 tbsp	Sesame seeds, dry roasted
1 tube	Wasabi (horseradish paste)
1 pkt	Pickled ginger (optional)
4 tbsp	Tamari
5 cups	Brown or basmati rice, cooked

Method

While the rice is still warm stir through the LSA and sesame seeds.

Let the rice sit while you prepare the other ingredients.

Peel the avocado and slice into strips.

Wash and separate the garlic chives.

Cut the cucumber into long thin strips.

Put the nori sheet on the sushi mat and cover the nori with a thin layer of rice.

Leave about 2cm (3/4 inch) clear at the top and bottom of the nori. Fill to the sides.

Spread a thin strip of wasabi along the center of the rice.

At the end closest to you, place 3 strips of garlic chives.

Put a strip of cucumber next then a strip of avocado.

Roll the mat up, away from you, creating a compact roll. Be careful not to roll the mat into the nori roll.

You can cut the long rolls into bite size pieces or just in half. Use a wet knife to do so.

Serve with pickled ginger, a dipping sauce of wasabi stirred into the tamari and a big green salad

Summer Chicken Kebabs - *Serves 4*
Something for the BBQ or under the grill on balmy summer nights.

4	*Chicken breast fillets, cut into bite sized pieces*
24	*Button mushrooms*
1 large	*Onion, cut into bite size pieces*
8	*Stainless steel or wooden skewers*

Marinade

1/3 cup	Cold pressed olive oil
2	Chillies, fresh finely sliced (optional)
2 tbsp	Coriander, fresh chopped
1 tsp	Ground turmeric
1 tsp	Ground cumin
2 tbsp	Tamari
1 tbsp	Lime or lemon juice

Method

Combine all marinade ingredients into a large bowl and stir well.

Add chicken pieces to marinade, cover and refrigerate for 2 hours.

When ready to cook, take a skewer and thread chicken, onion pieces and mushrooms alternately, until all 8 skewers are prepared

Barbecue, or grill, turning occasionally for 8 mins or until chicken is tender

Serve with your favorite summer salad

Alternatively you could replace the chicken with fish, lamb and/ or tofu!

Chicken Omelette - Serves 2

Ingredients

4 large	Eggs, free range
1 med	Zucchini, grated
1 cup	Chicken fillets, cut into thin strips
2 tbsp	Fish sauce
2 tsp	Sambal (chillies in vinegar), or fresh chili (optional)
1 cup	Chicken stock
1	Spring onion tops, chopped.
	Peanut or cold pressed olive oil for frying

Method

Use a frypan or wok.

Heat a small amount of the oil then quickly cook the chicken.

Once cooked, remove the chicken from the pan.

Crack the eggs and put into a mixing bowl.

Add the grated zucchini, strips of chicken and fish sauce into the bowl.

Whisk or beat the ingredients.

In the wok, place 1 tbsp oil, heat and swirl around.

Place half the ingredients and swirl around, flip over when brown.

Repeat for the other side.

Do exactly the same for the other omelette.

Heat the chicken stock.

Add 1 teaspoon of sambal (optional but delicious).

In 2 small bowls pour the chicken stock and sprinkle with spring onions.

Serve with a large side salad

Thai Green Chicken Curry - Serves 4

Ingredients

350g (12-13oz)	Chicken, chopped into pieces
1 tbsp	Thai green curry paste (you might like more)
1 tbsp	Cold pressed olive oil or coconut oil
1 cup	Green peas (fresh)
1 cup	Green beans, tipped and left whole
1 cup	Coconut cream
1/2 cup	Coriander

1 tbsp	Lemon, chopped very finely
2 whole	Red chillies (optional)
2 cups	Rice, cooked

Method

Heat oil in a pan on medium-low heat.

Add curry paste and heat for one minute.

Add half the coconut milk and cook until oil appears on the top.

Add chicken pieces and cook for around 10 minutes or until done.

Add the remaining coconut milk, green peas, beans and lemons.

Simmer until tender.

Garnish with sprigs of coriander.

Serve with boiled rice and fresh garden salad

Apricot Fat-Free Chicken - Serves 4

Ingredients

4 large	Chicken breast fillets, trimmed of all fat
4 tbsp	Dried apricots, chopped
2 tbsp	Hazelnuts, chopped
1 tsp	Dried oregano (if fresh, triple the amount and dice)
2	Garlic cloves, chopped

Sea salt and freshly ground black pepper to taste

Method

Mix apricots, nuts and oregano.

Cut the chicken fillets to open out as flat as possible.

Lay one fillet out and sprinkle 1/4 of filling over the flesh, repeat for the other 3 fillets.

Sprinkle top fillet with ground black pepper and a little oregano.

Tie fillets into a parcel shape with string and place into oven bag.

Add 2 tablespoons of apricot nectar or water to oven bag.

Bake in oven as directed - about 1 hour or until tender.

After cooking, snip bag and retain juices, make juices up to 1 cup with water, and use as a tasty sauce.

Slice your chicken parcel carefully with a sharp knife.

Fresh Fish with Ginger and Spring Onions - *Serves 4*

Tuna, Atlantic salmon or salmon trout are the preferred choices for this refreshing meal.

Try wrapping the fish in fresh banana leaves instead of foil. Available at Asian green grocers and in some supermarkets.

Ingredients

4 pieces	Fish of your choice, fresh
4 tsp	Cold pressed olive oil
3	Spring onions, sliced cross ways
1 piece	Ginger, freshly grated
4 pieces	Foil or banana leaves for wrapping fish
	Thinly sliced lemon wedges for garnish

Method

Preheat oven to 180 deg C or 350 deg F.

Place a piece of fish onto the foil or leaf.

Spoon over 1 teaspoon of oil, some ginger, spring onions and a lemon wedge.

Loosely cover with foil or wrap in banana leaves.

Repeat the process 3 more times for other pieces of fish.

Place all parcels in an oven proof dish.

Bake for 15 to 20 minutes.

When ready season with salt and pepper to taste.

Serve with a fresh cucumber salad.

Fish Steaks with Tangy Topping - Serves 4

Ingredients

Tangy topping can be served either hot or cold.

4	*White fish steaks*
2	*Tomatoes, seeded and chopped*
4	*Spring onions, chopped*
1 tbsp	*Basil, chopped*
2 tbsp	*Parsley, chopped*
1 tbsp	*Lemon juice*
1 tbsp	*Cold pressed olive oil*

Salt and ground black pepper to taste

Method

Cook fish under grill, 4 to 5 minutes each side. Keep warm until serving

Combine all other ingredients in bowl to make tomato mixture

Serve fish topped with tomato mixture, on a bed of rice or

noodles and a big green salad

Quick Beef and Mushroom Casserole - *Serves 4 - 6*

Ingredients

750g/27oz	Lean beef strips (rump is ideal)
1 large	Onion, cut into rings
1 tbsp	Cold pressed olive oil
1 med	Red capsicum, seeded and chopped
150g/5oz	Field mushrooms
2 cups	Water
2 tbsp	Tomato paste
2 tsp	Oregano, fresh and chopped

Method

Heat oil in large pan, brown beef, onion and capsicum, stir often.

Add all other ingredients, cover pan, Simmer for about 40 to 45 minutes.

Serve with rice, steamed carrots, snow peas and a big green salad.

Spicy Beef with Pulses - *Serves 4 or more*

Ingredients

500g/18oz	Premium fat free minced beef
3	Garlic cloves, crushed (more if desired)
1 large	Onion, chopped
420g/15oz	Tomatoes, canned, chopped
1 tsp	Chili (optional)
1 tsp	Turmeric
420g/15oz	Chick peas, canned, drained

1 tbsp   *Cold pressed olive oil*

Method

Heat oil in pan and brown meat.

Add onion and garlic, cook for 1 minute.

Add tomatoes, chili, turmeric and simmer until meat is tender.

Stir in chick peas until heated through.

Serve with a tossed green salad.

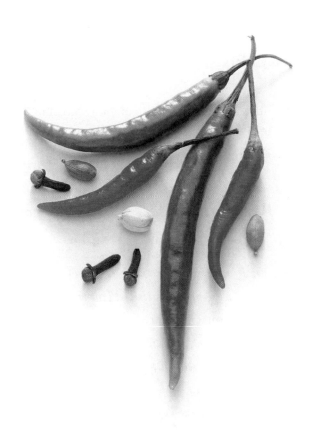

DESSERTS AND SWEET TREATS

Chia pudding

Ingredients

1 can of coconut milk

½ cup shredded coconut

4 tbsp chia seeds

2 tbsp raw honey or agave nectar

1 tsp cinnamon or cacao powder

1 tsp vanilla powder

Method

In a glass bowl add all the ingredients, then shake, shake, shake. Place in the fridge overnight or for at least 3 hours. Serve with fruit and a sprinkle of cinnamon. You can make these at night and have them for a delicious fiber filled breakfast or take them to work as a treat.

Chocolate and Date Balls

Ingredients

1 ¼ cup almond meal

¾ cup walnut meal

¼ cup raw cacao powder

1 tsp vanilla paste

1 tbsp chia seeds

1 tbsp linseed/flaxseed ground

Pinch of cinnamon

16 fresh dates

Method

Combine almond meal, walnut meal and cacao powder into a food processor and add the vanilla and dates. Process until mixture is combined. If the mixture is too dry and doesn't stick together add small amounts of water until the mixture is firm and sticky. Remove the mixture from the food processor into a bowl. Form into round balls and roll in a choice of coating (shredded coconut or cacao powder).

Lemon Cookies

Ingredients

400g shredded coconut

1 cup slivered almonds, chopped

½ cup coconut sugar

1 tsp vanilla paste

2 tsp grated lemon zest

4 large egg whites

Method

Preheat oven to 180C. Mix almonds, coconut, and sugar and lemon zest in a bowl and then mix in the egg whites gently. Drop dollops of mixture, equivalent to 2 tablespoons onto baking paper, keep them spaced out. Bake until the edges become brown, around 20 to 25min. Cool slightly then transfer onto a cooling rack.

Muesli Bars

Ingredients

1 cup rice bubbles

½ cup quinoa flakes

½ cup shredded coconut

1/3 cup chopped mixed nuts

1/3 cup cacao nibs

¼ cup pumpkin seeds

¼ cup sunflower seeds

2 Tbsp ground flax seed

2 Tbsp hemp seeds

¼ cup cold pressed organic coconut oil

½ cup almond butter

Method

Stir all the dry ingredients together thoroughly. Separately mix the wet ingredients together. Now combine both the mixtures and mix together well. Press into a lined baking tray. Chill in the fridge

Chocolate and Date Squares

Ingredients

2	*cups almond meal*
1	*cup macadamias, chopped*
2	*cups dates*
¾	*cup cacao powder*
¼	*tsp vanilla extract*
1	*tsp cold pressed coconut oil*
1	*tsp water*

Method

Roughly chop the dates. Place dates, macadamias, coconut oil and cacao powder into a food processor. Blend until completely smooth. Add the vanilla and small amount of water. Keep adding water until the paste is sticky. Press firmly into a lined pan and cover with alfoil. Refrigerate and once set, cut into desired sizes.

Chocolate and Orange Pudding

This recipe is so delicious even children will love it!

Ingredients

1/3	*cup raw or regular cocoa powder*
1	*cup pitted dates*
1	*vanilla bean, seeds scraped out (or 2 tsp pure vanilla extract)*
1	*cup roughly chopped ripe avocado (use around 1 large avocado)*
1	*tsp orange zest (zest orange before juicing it)*
1/2	*cup fresh squeezed orange juice*
1/8 tsp	*salt*

Method

Puree all ingredients in a food processor until very, very smooth. This pudding is very thick and if desired you can add more orange juice, a dash of coconut or almond milk. Pour into plastic cups and refrigerate covered.

Coconut Bread

Mildly sweet and light bread

Ingredients

3/4	*cup coconut flour*
1/2	*cup butter*
6	*eggs, whole*
1-2	*tablespoon honey, depending on taste*

1/2 teaspoon salt

1 teaspoon baking powder

Method

Preheat oven to 180°C (350°F). Blend all ingredients in a food processor until all lumps are gone. Grease a bread pan and pour in batter in. Bake for 40 minutes.

Lemon Cheesecake Bars

Yield: makes 16 (2-inch x 2-inch) squares

Crust Ingredients

4	*dates, pitted*
1	*cup raw pecans*
1/2	*cup walnuts*
1	*tablespoon coconut oil*
3/4	*teaspoon ginger root powder or cinnamon powder*
¼ tsp	*salt*

Cheesecake Filling Ingredients

1 1/2	*cups raw cashews, soaked*
¼	*cup dairy milk or coconut milk*
¼	*cup fresh squeezed lemon juice*
2 tbsp	*butter – dairy*
2 tbsp	*coconut oil*
2 tbsp	*raw honey*
1 tbsp	*vanilla extract*
zest from one lemon	
pinch of salt	

To make the crust

Line a baking tray with parchment paper.

Put the pecans and walnuts in a powerful blender. Pulse several times to break up the nuts. Add dates, salt, coconut oil and ground ginger root or cinnamon powder. Blend until the mixture begins to come together as a dough.

Press the nut mixture evenly into the bottom of the lined pan. Set aside.

To make the filling

- Put the cashews, milk, lemon juice, butter, coconut oil, honey, vanilla extract, lemon zest, and salt into a high-powered blender. Start on low, gradually increase to high and process until completely smooth.

- Add this mixture on top of the crust and smooth over the top. Cover and place in the freezer for at least 6 hours.

- Leave at room temperature for 15 to 20 minutes before cutting and serving.

- Caution: Don't let this dessert sit at room temperature for too long or it will get very soft. It's best when served chilled.

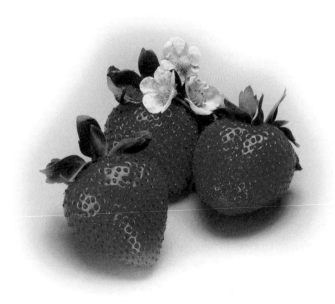

Processed Gluten Free Foods

Studies have shown that gluten free processed diet products may not be good sources of minerals (such as iron, zinc, magnesium, iodine and selenium), or vitamins (such as folate, B vitamins and vitamin E) and the nutritional content of gluten-free foods can be a problem if they form a large part of the diet.

Studies have shown that patients with gluten intolerance have inadequate intake of minerals (magnesium, calcium, iron, zinc and selenium) and folate, thiamine, vitamin A and fiber compared with people who are not gluten intolerant.

Previous studies have shown that processed gluten-free products have high levels of cheap processed fats (trans fats) and refined sugars. Individuals with Celiac Disease generally compensate for their restricted diet by eating pre-packaged processed gluten free foods containing high levels of trans fat, sugar and calories, therefore gluten intolerant patients may become overweight

If you are following a gluten free diet it is important to include a lot of unprocessed foods that are not in a packet. Gluten-free whole grains such as quinoa, amaranth, millet and teff contain more minerals, vitamins, fiber and antioxidants than wheat.

New developments under way

Vaccine against gluten intolerance

There is an exciting new treatment being developed in Australia which may be able to cure Celiac Disease. This treatment, known as a Therapeutic Peptide Vaccine, helps to modulate and change the immune system of people with Celiac Disease by changing the way their body reacts to gluten. By stopping the immune reaction to gluten, this vaccine is able to prevent the inflammatory reaction which occurs in the gut. It is believed that the vaccination will be prescribed in conjunction with a gluten free diet, however if it is found to be efficacious it may replace gluten free dieting for Celiacs all together.

New ways of testing for Celiac Disease are also being developed. By testing key genetic markers of potential Celiac Disease sufferers researchers were able to determine those people who were at genetic risk of gluten allergy without the hassle of a bowel biopsy.

Enzymes to digest gluten

Enzymes are found in the digestive tract all the way from the mouth to the large intestine. They are responsible for breaking down foods so they are able to be absorbed from the gut and into our bloodstream. Often people who are gluten sensitive have lower amounts of gluten digesting enzymes in their digestive tract. Digestion of gluten begins in the stomach after being mixed with hydrochloric acid (HCL)) and pepsinogen. After this, the protein containing foods are moved through into the small intestine, where pancreatic enzymes, trypsin and chymotrypsin, finish the digestive process.

Do gluten digesting enzymes work?

We do get questions regarding the use of enzymes that are marketed to digest gluten.

Are the enzyme supplements safe? Do they work? Is there any risk from using these enzymes? Gluten digestive enzyme products on the market today include GlutenEase, Gluten Digest, Gluten Freeze and more. Many variations of these enzyme products are being offered, and people are trying them.

The truth is that none of these products has undergone clinical trials or testing to determine their efficacy and safety in people with Celiac Disease and non-celiac gluten sensitivity (NCGS).

What do the experts say?

Leading celiac experts agree that the enzyme supplements currently on the market digest only a tiny number of gluten molecules, which makes them unsafe for people with Celiac Disease and non-celiac gluten sensitivity.

We have seen patients with Celiac Disease use these enzyme supplements as a bandaid to consume gluten. Although most of the products state on the label that they are not safe for people with Celiac Disease, many ignore that disclaimer. Thus some celiac patients rely on these enzymes to have "just a taste" of something containing gluten. People with true gluten intolerance learn quickly that these products don't work for them.

If you have Celiac Disease, damage from gluten ingestion can occur regardless of whether you are aware of any symptoms. These supplements are not tested for celiac patients or those with NCGS and should be avoided by them no matter how mild or severe their symptoms.

People are worried about parties, holidays, cross contamination with gluten and whether there is any way for them to tolerate "just a little bit" of gluten. Our answer is no.

Are gluten digesting enzymes effective or safe for patients with non-celiac gluten sensitivity (NCGS)?

The answer is, we really do not know. We still have so much to learn about gluten sensitivity. There are no scientific studies looking at the efficacy and safety of these enzyme products in gluten-sensitive patients. Without scientific evidence, we do not know whether these products are safe or useful.

Some of these enzyme supplements have other things added such as probiotics, vitamins and minerals in which gluten intolerant patients are often deficient. These additional components may make you feel better, and not the enzyme component.

Gluten digesting enzymes are not the miracle pill or panacea we all are hoping for. However there are other products in major clinical trials that look quite positive for pharmaceutical treatments for Celiac Disease and gluten sensitivity.

Summary

So in summary hidden gluten intolerance could be the reason you are not as healthy as you should be. In gluten intolerant people there is a genetic predisposition for gluten to cause excess inflammation which can manifest anywhere in the body. Gluten may be the trigger that turns on the wrong genes in your DNA (genome) and this can cause an autoimmune problem to begin or become worse.

Autoimmune problems can vary widely

Thyroid conditions such as Hashimoto's Thyroiditis or Grave's disease.

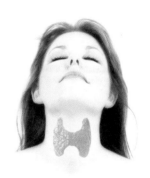

Thyroid problems are incredibly common but very few doctors know that gluten can be a trigger for these problems and make them persist despite conventional treatment. Gluten can also cause your thyroid hormone tablets not to work. This is because the gluten primes your immune cells to make excessive amounts of thyroid antibodies that attack your thyroid gland. If you avoid gluten and take a selenium supplement you will see these antibodies come down – hooray – your thyroid tissue is no longer being destroyed. Gluten can also upset liver function, so that your liver and muscles do not convert thyroid hormone (thyroxine or T 4) into the much more active form of thyroid hormone (triiodothyronine or T 3). It can also cause your liver to make the wrong shape of T 3, which does not work at all.

Skin conditions such as dermatitis, psoriasis or dermatitis herpetiformis.

These skin problems are caused or greatly aggravated by dietary gluten. All the steroids and immune-suppressant drugs will not work for long or not work very well if you have a dysfunctional gut, liver and immune system caused by gluten.

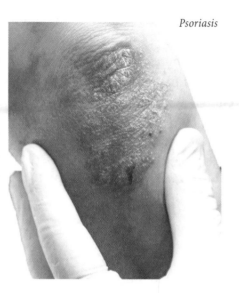

Psoriasis

Inflammatory disease of the intestines

These include gastritis, Crohn's Disease, Ulcerative Colitis and collagenous colitis. Of course the classic case is Celiac Disease where the small intestine is severely damaged so that malnutrition occurs.

Pernicious anemia causing severe deficiency of Vitamin B 12

Here gluten causes the genes to make antibodies that attack the lining of the stomach so that you cannot make the essential factor produced in the stomach to absorb vitamin B 12. This can cause depression, fatigue and nerve damage.

Multiple sclerosis

It is not widely recognized that gluten can cause severe inflammation in the central nervous system (the brain), spine and the peripheral nerves. If you have MS, go gluten free.

Gluten induced ataxia

In this condition gluten causes damage to the part of the brain called the cerebellum. The cerebellum controls and coordinates limb movements so that you have a normal gait and do not become clumsy or fall over. In gluten induced ataxia the gait becomes clumsy and the legs are wider apart when walking – you walk like someone who is drunk and will have frequent falls. This condition is not uncommon in children.

Liver disease

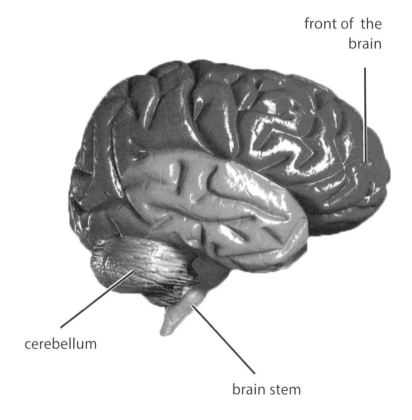

front of the brain

cerebellum

brain stem

Some types of liver diseases are triggered by gluten causing inflammation in various parts of the liver. This inflammation can aggravate autoimmune hepatitis, Primary Biliary Cirrhosis (PBC) and Sclerosing Cholangitis.

Arteritis (inflammation of the blood vessels known as

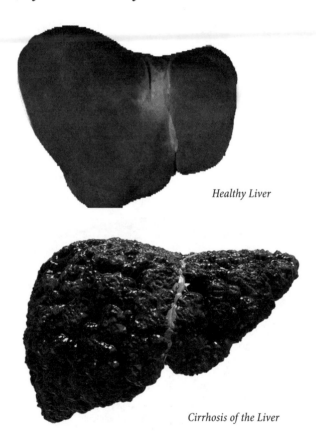

Healthy Liver

Cirrhosis of the Liver

arteries)

This can occur in blood vessels in any part of the body, including the brain when it can cause headaches, cognitive impairment or strokes. It is not uncommon for over vaccination or antibiotic use to trigger arteritis in a gluten intolerant person.

Systemic Lupus Erythematosis (SLE)

SLE is a condition where the immune system makes antibodies that attack the inner most part of the cells (the cell nucleus and its contained DNA). It can vary from mild and skin based or it can aggressively attack any part of your body. It is imperative to follow a gluten free diet and take selenium.

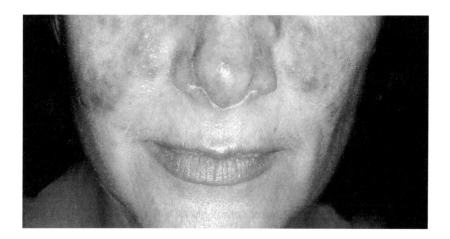

Polymyalgia Rheumatica and Fibromyalgia

These are painful conditions affecting the connective tissues (skeletal muscles and tendons). In Polymyalgia Rheumatica the onset of the pain is sudden and the pain is severe and often immobilizing. It can affect the muscles and tendons in the neck, back, arms, pelvic girdle and legs. The muscles are so inflamed that they are "cooked" and it can be agony. Steroids are always required. Fibromyalgia is a similar type of pain but much mush less severe and is usually chronic. A gluten free diet is imperative. Supplements of magnesium, vitamin D, selenium and omega 3 are required.

Arthritis and tendinitis

Some forms of arthritis, from rheumatoid, psoriatic to

osteoarthritis, are surely worsened by eating gluten. Tendinitis such as plantar fasciitis, RSI and Achilles tendinitis can be aggravated by gluten.

Eye conditions

Autoimmune eye conditions such as iritis (inflammation of the colored iris) and scleritis (inflammation of the whites of the eyes) and ulcers on the front of the eye can be triggered or aggravated by gluten. I have had several patients who were completely cured of iritis and corneal ulcers by following a gluten free diet and taking antioxidants and selenium

Many more types of autoimmune disease and so called "mysterious inflammatory problems" can be caused by gluten and its associated nutritional deficiencies.

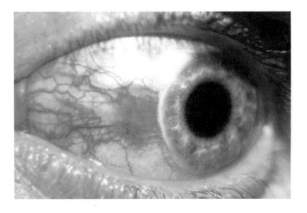

Scleritis

Gluten and inflammation

Gluten can cause:

- Full-blown Celiac Disease is an autoimmune disease that triggers severe inflammation in the small intestines. Gluten can also cause widespread inflammation in the body which can cause conditions including autoimmune diseases, cancer, depression, osteoporosis and more.

- Whole body inflammation — a NON-gluten glycoprotein or lectin (this is a complex of sugar and protein) present in wheat is called wheat germ agglutinin (WGA). WGA can trigger whole body inflammation. This is not technically an autoimmune reaction but it can still cause severe health problems.

- Less severe inflammatory reactions to gluten trigger the same problems even if you don't have diagnosed Celiac Disease, but you only have elevated antibodies (7% of the population has these elevated levels of anti-gliadin antibodies). These antibodies were also found in 18% of people with autism and 20% of those with schizophrenia.

The modern day dwarf wheat or FrankenWheat contains super gluten which is much more likely to create inflammation in the body.

The vast majority of people with an autoimmune disease have a "leaky gut", which is an excessively permeable gut or intestine. It is vital to heal a leaky gut if you have an autoimmune disease.

Dr. Alessio Fasano, a celiac expert from the University of Maryland discovered a protein made in the intestines called "zonulin." Interestingly zonulin production is increased by exposure to gluten. Excess zonulin is not good, as it breaks up the tight junctions (cement) between the intestinal cells. These tight junctions prevent bacteria, toxins and foreign proteins in food leaking across the intestinal barrier into the bloodstream.

Gluten is a protein found in wheat, barley, rye, spelt and oats. Gluten may cause Celiac Disease only, or it may provoke severe inflammation throughout the body; it has been linked to many autoimmune diseases, mood disorders, mental illness such as bipolar and schizophrenia, neuro-degenerative diseases (such as multiple sclerosis and dementia), autism and cancer.

The problems with gluten are very real and scientifically validated and yet many doctors are not interested or have a closed mind. Eliminating gluten may not only make you feel more energetic and lose weight, it could save your life.

Gluten intolerance may not be the only cause of autoimmune diseases; however gluten can act to trigger or exacerbate latent or existing autoimmune diseases.

The nutritional deficiencies caused by gluten intolerance also make the inflammation of autoimmune diseases much worse and necessitate a larger dose of anti-inflammatory supplements such as vitamin D, vitamin K 2, omega 3 fatty acids, vitamin C, zinc and selenium.

In people with excessive inflammation and gluten intolerance we must improve the health of the gut and the liver and reduce inflammation in these areas. A good probiotic supplement and eating fermented foods can improve the health of the gut.

The liver function can be improved by eating more vegetables, both cooked and raw, and by raw vegetable juicing. I also advise taking a good liver formula such as Livatone Plus to support the healthy function of the liver. The liver protects the immune system from overload and toxicity because of its ability to break down toxins. The liver is the filter and cleanser of the bloodstream and can remove immune complexes caused by gluten and other allergens. If the liver filter does not remove these complexes they will circulate in the bloodstream leading to inflammation and possibly autoimmune diseases.

Over the last decade a much wider range of gluten-related

illnesses has become recognized by immunologists and researchers. This includes a category characterized by NOT being consistent with the well-documented tests and markers for autoimmune Celiac Disease, gluten allergy or wheat allergy. One must have a high degree of awareness that gluten could be the hidden factor, if typical symptoms persist even though all tests are negative.

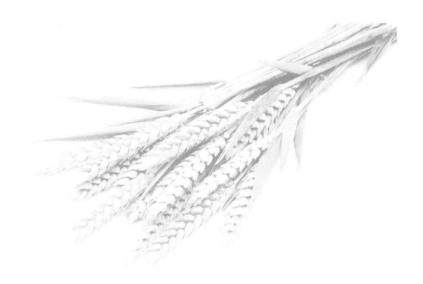

Beneficial Fermented Foods for the Digestive Tract

Fermented foods are extremely beneficial because they produce a more favorable population of bacteria in the intestines. This is imperative for gluten intolerant people to heal and keep their gut healthy.

Fermented foods contain trillions of beneficial bacteria (probiotics) compared to probiotic supplements which usually contain several billion to 30 billion per serve. Fermented foods provide a wider diversity of probiotics than probiotic supplements do. Fermented foods are a potent way to use food to add to the diversity of good species (micro-organisms) inhabiting our digestive system.

Fermented foods can reduce many types of chronic digestive and bowel symptoms and even overcome autoimmune diseases, especially if a gluten free diet is followed and the correct supplements are taken. Normal gut flora has more than 600 different species and most available commercial probiotic products contain a maximum of nine species. After any course of antibiotics it is necessary to repopulate our intestine with as wide a variety of healthy micro organisms as possible. Many people with chronic digestive and bowel problems have a host of bad species in their gut and not enough good or healthy species (probiotics). Until this is reversed you cannot restore your health.

Dairy sourced

Yoghurt – purchase full fat, unsweetened, unflavored and preferably organic or biodynamic. This type of yogurt may be purchased or made at home by using prepared yogurt as the starter or a commercial product like EasyYo or Progurt may be used. Avoid the sweetened choices, as sugar kills the probiotics.

Kefir – is cultured probiotic milk; it's easy to make at home from commercially available freeze dried granules, which are available from health stores.

Cheese – Camembert, Brie and moldy cheeses are fermented. Always buy these fresh and do not allow them to age for too long.

Normal cheeses do not use probiotics in their manufacture.

Crème fraiche - is cultured cream. After being seeded with probiotics it is cultured for 3 - 4 days before being churned. This process results in resulting in both probiotic rich butter and real buttermilk.

Cultured buttermilk – is the liquid portion of the butter churning process. It may be flavored with berries, coffee or vanilla and some stevia drops to make a probiotic rich drinking yogurt. It is often used in flap jacks, but the cooking kills the beneficial bacteria.

Vegetable sourced

Sauerkraut – traditional European winter food. It is cabbage based with other available vegetables added, then salted and naturally fermented with fresh liquid whey from either aged yogurt or kefir.

Kalekraut – is very similar to Sauerkraut but is made with kale instead of cabbage. It is made the same way and the resultant product tends to be less sour in flavor.

Kim Chi – is the national dish of Korea and is made in a similar way to sauerkraut with the addition of many other vegetables, spices and especially chili. It also tends to be quite highly salted and many types have added salted fish.

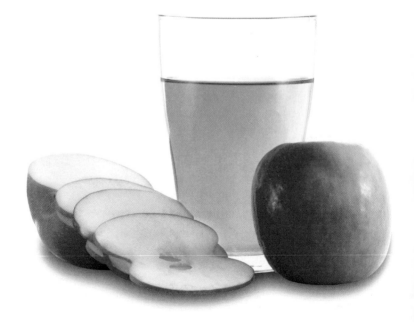

Fermented Vegetable Recipe

Mauritian Cabbage Pickle

½ a firm cabbage, finely sliced.

3 carrots, julienned.

¼ pound fresh green beans, thinly sliced.

Other vegetables in season may be added to your taste.

Place the vegetables in the sun in a thin layer to partially dehydrate.

Meanwhile

2 onions thinly sliced lengthways, gently fried in 3 tablespoons of virgin coconut oil.

Add 3cm fresh ginger, grated.

1 whole garlic onion; peeled and passed through presser.

1 teaspoon freshly ground black pepper

1 tablespoon turmeric, depending on taste.

1 tablespoon white mustard seed and gently heat this mixture

til turmeric becomes dark in colour.

Turn off heat and add the sliced vegetables.

Add ¼ cup of cold pressed extra virgin olive oil and apple cider vinegar (with the mother).

Celtic sea salt may also be added to taste.

The pickle is ready for use and is best stored in the refrigerator and improves with age.

Soy or Rice Sourced

Natto – definitely not for the feint hearted. This food is eaten with gusto in Japan but in western countries it has not gained the same popularity. Natto is soy beans that have been fermented with a bacteria and the product is distinctive in both taste and appearance.

Miso – is a fermented product of soy or barley or rice. Some brands have a mixture of these, which makes it a gluten free or very low gluten product. Miso may be enjoyed as a meal starter or soup and may be added to meals to impart a distinctive salty-sweet flavor and beneficial nutrients.

Tempeh - is blocks of soy bean that have been fermented with a beneficial fungus. It may be sliced and added to salads or stir fried and used in the same way as tofu.

Plant Sourced

Kombucha Tea – requires sweetened tea for the growth of this probiotic rich drink. It is made by adding a kombucha starter to cooled sweetened tea and left to ferment at room temperature until sweetness is replaced by a more acidic taste.

Vinegar – is probably our best known household fermented food and it is produced from the fermentation of wines, fruits or flowers. Inferior vinegars are simply diluted acetic acid and are definitely not a healthy alternative. These are often simply identified as white vinegar or malt vinegar.

Apple cider vinegar – is easily purchased and the best probiotic value is found in a product with a 'mother'. The mother is sediment on the bottom of the bottle and this provides a rich source of probiotic.

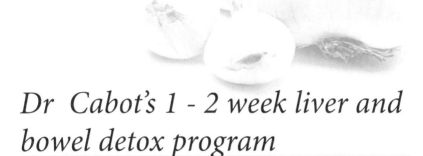

Dr Cabot's 1 - 2 week liver and bowel detox program

A deep quick cleanse for Gluten Intolerant people

Today we cannot escape environmental toxins as they are increasingly in the air, water, soil and by extension, in the food we eat. Of course we can always grow some of our own food if we are lucky enough to have a backyard and use natural compost and fertilizers and I highly recommend this. Probably the most toxic thing that is happening to our planet is coal gas seam mining and horizontal drilling which is literally flooding our underground water channels with thousands of toxic chemicals. This is a good reason to install a rain water tank. As the North American Indians said about the white man, "Only when the last fish is poisoned will man realize that he cannot eat money"

So what can we do to reduce our body's chemical load?

The liver is the only organ that can breakdown (metabolize) fat soluble toxins and turn them into water soluble forms. Once they are water soluble they can be eliminated via the watery fluids of the body such as the bile, sweat, saliva and urine. If you liver does not break them down they will stay in the fatty parts of your body, which is not a good situation for your immune system or your metabolism. Toxic chemical overload can lead to weight gain and this is why a 1 to 2 week detox can promote weight loss as well as better energy levels.

Here are the principles of the program –

- Drink 10 glasses of water daily – drink it throughout the day
- Start the day with a glass of water containing the juice of a freshly squeezed lemon or lime

Eat only the following during your 1 to 2 week detox –

Fruits and vegetables - the fruits and vegetables can be raw and cooked. You may have any vegetable you want including starchy vegetables such as sweet potato, carrot, parsnips and turnips etc. If you make a vegetable soup, use may use vegetable stock, Herbamare or miso to flavor it. To cook the vegetables, you may use the following methods - steam them, roast them or stir fry them with olive oil. You can spread or paste the vegetables with a thin layer of olive oil or coconut oil before you roast them in the oven. Do not use a microwave oven to cook your vegetables or fruits, as this is irradiating your food and will damage the cell structures in the vegetables and fruits. You can stew the fruits in their own juice and water with a tiny amount of honey or stevia. Cinnamon sticks add a nice flavor to stewed fruits. If you can afford it, purchase organic fruits and vegetables.

Salad dressing ingredients – you may use cold pressed olive oil or macadamia oil, coconut oil, apple cider vinegar, mustard, fresh lemon or lime and fresh or dried herbs. Mix ingredients in a jar and shake or whisk with a fork or blend in a blender

Raw nuts and seeds – you can choose any seeds (pumpkin seeds, hemp seeds, chia seeds, ground flaxseeds) and any raw nuts

Tahini and hummus are allowed and make a nice dip with avocado and lemon

Milks – only coconut or almond milk is allowed

Drink 8 ounces to 10 ounces (250 to 300mls) of raw juice daily – best ingredients to juice are parsley, basil, mint, carrot, cabbage, beet, green apple, lemon, orange and ginger. You can also add a cruciferous vegetable to the juice such as kale, broccoli, Brussels sprouts or cauliflower.

Take a powerful liver tonic such as containing the herb Milk Thistle, Turmeric, B vitamins and the amino acid Taurine and Selenium to support the detoxification process in your liver.

www.seleniumresearch.com

Super foods to detox

- Garlic and fresh ginger
- Curry and/or Turmeric
- Broccoli sprouts powder or capsules
- Glutamine powder heals a leaky gut
- Tahini paste
- Organic apple cider vinegar

You may want to do this detox diet several times during a year to keep your total body toxin level at acceptable levels.

Suggested supplements during your Detox

FibreTone Powder 2 teaspoons daily in water, coconut milk or raw juices

Livatone Plus two capsules twice daily

Glutamine Powder – 1 tsp twice daily in a cool beverage such as coconut, almond or rice milk

How do you know if you need a Detox?

Look at your tongue – is it coated or discolored?

Do you have constipation and/or abdominal bloating?

Do you have Fatty liver?

Do you have excessive weight?

Do you have allergies and/or skin rashes?

Do you have frequent headaches?

Do you take a lot of pain killers?

Do you have recurrent sinus infections?

How are allergies mediated in the body?

The word mediated means the mechanism by which something is produced and transmitted in the body

IgE-Mediated Food Allergy

IgE is a protein (immunoglobulin) made by the cells of the immune system. The level of IgE in the blood is abnormally high in very allergic people. A classic example of IgE-mediated food allergy occurs in someone who is allergic to a food (especially nuts or shell fish) and who has an obvious allergic reaction within minutes of eating a small (sometimes extremely tiny) amount of the offending food.

This type of allergic reaction is caused by the allergen (eg.nut or shellfish) reacting with IgE, which produces an explosive release of histamine. The reaction occurs over minutes (or occasionally several hours); this causes symptoms such as itching, hives and swelling of the throat and eyes, runny nose, sneezing, wheezing, coughing, vomiting or diarrhea. Sometimes changes in blood pressure may be produced as part of this type of allergic reaction. IgE mediated food allergies are more likely to be life threatening and these people require to carry adrenalin injections (Epi-pen) on their person. This is the only way to abort a severe allergic reaction which could progress to anaphylaxis.

Non-IgE-mediated reactions

Allergies that are not caused by IgE antibodies are typically slower in onset and produce symptoms over hours to days after exposure to the food allergen. The symptoms are most commonly in the gastrointestinal system and include diarrhea, gas and cramps. Rashes that are itchy and red may also occur as well as headaches and sinus congestion. The allergic symptoms disappear after the food is removed from the diet. This may take a few weeks.

Elevated levels of IgE antibodies in the blood will not be found. The delay in the onset of symptoms following ingestion of the food allergen can makes it harder to identify the offending food or foods.

Celiac disease is an example of a non-IgE mediated gastrointestinal reaction to a food. Celiac disease is due to a sensitivity to gluten (gliadin) and this damage is slowly mediated, as contrasted with quickly produced IgE mediated allergies.

In those with Celiac Disease, gluten causes a much slower allergic reaction, which gradually damages the cells lining the small intestine. This damage causes bloating, abdominal pain, diarrhea and appetite changes. Severe weight loss may also occur. In children Celiac Disease produces failure to thrive.

As you can see the way allergies, sensitivities and intolerances are produced in the body is very complex and the field of immunology is a fascinating one to study. The varied ways in which people can react to gluten often makes it harder to get a clear diagnosis. Furthermore allergies and intolerances to several different foods often co-exist. This is why a detox may be a good idea – see page 88

In summary gluten intolerance may be mediated in different ways such as -

- **Immune-mediated reactions** causing symptoms from hours to several days after eating gluten. Typical symptoms produced are often similar to Celiac Disease symptoms. The blood tests and bowel biopsies do not show the distinctive autoimmune markers of Celiac Disease. Thus it is not Celiac Disease but is Non Celiac Gluten Sensitivity (NCGS)

- **Autoimmune reactions** causing Celiac Disease or other autoimmune diseases associated with Celiac Disease such as dermatitis herpetiformis. The intolerance manifests symptoms from weeks to years after gluten exposure

- **Allergic reactions** (with onset of symptoms within minutes to hours after gluten exposure). This is often an allergy to wheat and these are usually IgE mediated and often show elevated IgE antibiodies in the blood.

References

Saja K, Chatterjee U, Chatterjee BP, Sudhakaran PR. *Activation dependent expression of MMPs in peripheral blood mononuclear cells involves protein kinase A. Mol Cell Biochem. 2007 Feb;296(1-2):185-92.*

Dalla Pellegrina C, Perbellini O, et al. *Effects of wheat germ agglutinin on human gastrointestinal epithelium: insights experimental model of immune/epithelial cell interaction. Toxicol Appl Pharmacol. 2009 Jun 1;237(2):146-53.*

Rubio-Tapia A, Kyle RA, et al. *Increased prevalence and mortality in undiagnosed Celiac Disease. Gastroenterology. 2009 Jul;137(1):88-93.*

Ludvigsson JF, Montgomery SM, et al. *Small-intestinal histopathology and mortality risk in Celiac Disease. JAMA. 2009 Sep 16;302(11):1171-8.*

Fasano A. *Physiological, pathological, and therapeutic implications of zonulin-mediated intestinal barrier modulation: living life on the edge of the wall. Am J Pathol. 2008 Nov;173(5):1243-52.*

Marios Hadjivassiliou, et al. *Gluten ataxia in perspective: epidemiology, genetic susceptibility and clinical characteristics Brain. 2003 Mar;126(Pt 3):685-91*

Shor D.B. et al. *Gluten sensitivity in multiple sclerosis: experimental myth or clinical truth? Annals of the New York Academy of Sciences. 2009 Sep;1173:343-9*

Chin Lye Ch'ng, et al. *Celiac disease and autoimmune thyroid disease. Clinical Medicine and Research. October 1, 2007 vol. 5 no. 3 184-192*

Bhatia BK et al. *Diet and psoriasis, part II: Celiac disease and role of a gluten-free diet. J Am Acad Dermatol. 2014 Apr 26. pii: S0190-9622(14)01244-4*

Biesiekierski JR, et al. *Gluten Causes Gastrointestinal Symptoms in Subjects Without Celiac Disease: A Double-Blind Randomized Placebo-Controlled Trial. Am J Gastroenterol. 2011 Jan 11*

(Gluten causes increased gut permeability in celiacs and non celiacs): Sandro Drago, et al. *Gliadin, zonulin and gut permeability: Effects on celiac and non-celiac intestinal mucosa and intestinal cell lines. Scand J Gastroenterol. 2006 Apr;41(4):408-19.*

www.celiac.org.au

www.cyrexlabs.com/CyrexTestsArrays/tabid/136/Default.aspx - Gluten intolerance testing

Books by Sandra Cabot MD

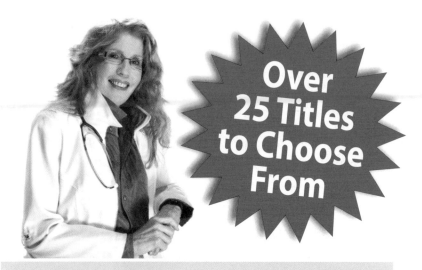

Over 25 Titles to Choose From

Titles by Sandra Cabot MD

Alzheimer's - What you must know to protect your brain and improve your memory

Bird Flu - Your Personal Survival Guide

The Body Shaping Diet - Discover your body type

Boost Your Energy

Breast Cancer Prevention Guide

Can't Lose Weight? You Could Have Syndrome X

Cholesterol: The Real Truth - are the drugs you take making you sick?

Diabetes Type 2: You Can Reverse It Naturally

Endometriosis Your Best Chance To Cure It (eBook only)

Fatty Liver: You Can Reverse It

Healthy Bowel Healthy Body - an A to Z Guide to Heal the Bowel

Help For Depression and Anxiety

Increase Your Sex Drive Naturally

Infertility: The Hidden Causes How to overcome them naturally

Low Carb Cocktail Party - created with all natural ingredients

Hormones - Don't Let Them Ruin Your Life

Hormone Replacement - The Real Truth - Bioidentical hormones

How Not To Kill Your Husband

The Liver Cleansing Diet

Magnesium the Miracle Mineral - You won't believe the difference it makes to your health and your sex life

Raw Juices Can Save Your Life - An A to Z guide for diseases

Save Your Gallbladder Naturally and what to do if you've already lost it

Tired of Not Sleeping? - Holistic program for a good night's sleep

The Ultimate Detox

Want to Lose Weight, But Hooked On Food?

Your Thyroid Problems Solved